Dr. Martinelli's Modern Glaucoma

Practical Insights and Emerging Trends in Glaucoma Care

The Fine Art of Patient Management

John R Martinelli MD OD FAAO

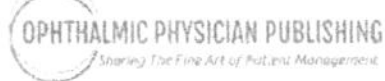

OPHTHALMIC PHYSICIAN PUBLISHING
Sharing The Fine Art of Patient Management

For Melissa,

Your patience, love, and encouragement
have made this book possible.

I am forever grateful.

Medical Disclaimer

Please note the information contained within this book is for educational purposes only. All effort has been executed to present accurate, up-to-date, reliable, complete information. The content within this book has been derived from various sources. Please consult a licensed physician before implementing diagnostic methods and/or treatments outlined in this book.

By reading this book, the reader agrees that under no circumstances is the author responsible for any losses, direct or indirect, that are incurred because of the use of the information contained within this book, including, but not limited to, errors, omissions, or inaccuracies.

Please note the information provided below is for general informational purposes. It is not intended to diagnose, treat, cure, or prevent any disease, and it should not be relied upon as a substitute for consultations with qualified healthcare professionals.

Ophthalmic Physician Publishing strives to ensure the information presented is accurate and up to date, but we make no representations or warranties of any kind, express or implied, about the completeness, accuracy, reliability, suitability, or availability with respect to the information provided. Any reliance you place on such information is strictly at your own risk.

Contents

Chapter 1

The Landscape of Glaucoma

Glaucoma is a complex and heterogeneous group of optic neuropathies characterized by the progressive degeneration of retinal ganglion cells and their axons, potentially leading to irreversible vision loss. It is one of the leading causes of vision loss globally, affecting over 70 million individuals, with nearly 10% of those cases becoming bilateral. The multifactorial nature of glaucoma presents significant challenges in its diagnosis, management, and treatment, necessitating a comprehensive understanding of its pathophysiology, risk factors, and clinical manifestations.

History

The understanding of glaucoma has evolved significantly over centuries. Early descriptions of the condition date back to ancient Greek medicine, where it was often conflated with cataracts under the term *"glaukos,"* which referred to a blue-green discoloration of the eye.

It wasn't until the 19th century that glaucoma began to be distinguished as a distinct entity, primarily through the work of pioneering ophthalmologists like Albrecht von Graefe, who linked elevated intraocular pressure (IOP) with optic nerve damage.

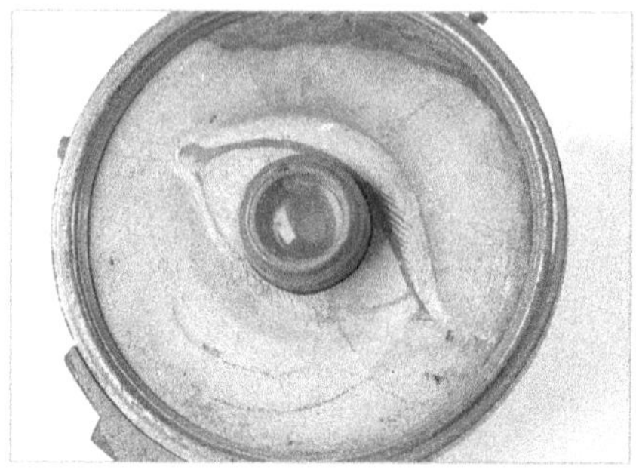

Model eye, glass lens and brass-backed paper front with hand-painted face around eye, by W. & S. Jones, London 1840-1900, Wellcome Images

Epidemiology: Global & Regional Prevalence

The global burden of glaucoma is substantial, with its prevalence varying significantly across different populations and geographic regions. *Primary open-angle glaucoma (POAG) is the most common form*, accounting for approximately 74% of all glaucoma cases worldwide. The prevalence of POAG is highest in African and Caribbean populations, where the condition tends to present earlier, and progress more rapidly compared to other ethnic groups. This heightened susceptibility is thought to be related to both genetic and environmental factors, though the exact mechanisms remain incompletely understood.

In contrast, *primary angle-closure glaucoma (PACG) is more prevalent in Asian populations*, particularly among individuals of Chinese and Southeast Asian descent. PACG is associated with anatomic predispositions such as a shallow anterior chamber and a narrow angle, which increase the risk of angle closure and subsequent IOP elevation. This form of glaucoma is less common in Western populations but tends to be more severe when it does occur, often requiring prompt surgical intervention to prevent vision loss.

The global prevalence of glaucoma is expected to increase as the population ages, with projections suggesting that the number of affected individuals will rise to over 111 million by 2040. This anticipated increase underscores the urgent need for improved screening, early detection, and effective management strategies, particularly in low and middle-income countries where access to eye care services may be limited.

Economic & Social Impact of Glaucoma

Glaucoma imposes a significant economic burden on both individuals and healthcare systems. The direct costs associated with glaucoma include expenses related to diagnosis, ongoing management, medical and surgical treatments, and medications. Indirect costs, such as lost productivity due to visual impairment and the need for caregiver support, further exacerbate the financial impact of the condition.

In high-income countries, the costs of glaucoma care are substantial and continue to rise as the population ages and new, often expensive, treatment modalities are introduced. For example, the annual cost of managing glaucoma in the *United States is estimated to exceed $2.5 billion, with an average lifetime cost per patient of approximately $16,000.* These figures do not account for the additional economic burden of indirect costs, which can be particularly devastating for individuals and families in low and middle-income countries where healthcare resources are scarce and out-of-pocket expenses are high.

Beyond the economic impact, glaucoma also has profound social and psychological consequences. Vision loss from glaucoma can lead to less independence, reduced quality of life, and increased risk of depression and anxiety. The fear of losing vision, coupled with the chronic nature of the condition and need for lifelong treatment, can also contribute to a significant psychological burden for individuals. Addressing these issues requires a holistic approach to glaucoma care that encompasses not only medical and surgical management but also psychosocial support and patient education.

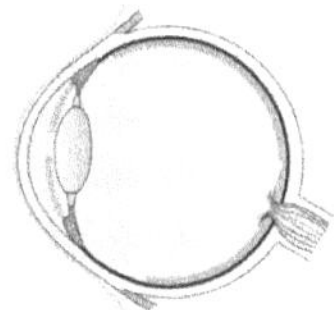

Chapter 2
Relative Anatomy

Glaucoma, a group of optic neuropathies, is characterized by *progressive degeneration of retinal ganglion cells* (RGCs) and their axons, leading to irreversible vision loss. The condition primarily affects the anterior visual pathways, including the retina, optic nerve, and optic tracts, but its impact extends to the visual cortex, which processes visual information. Understanding the detailed anatomy and physiology of these structures is critical for comprehending the pathogenesis of glaucoma and the resulting visual deficits.

Retina

The human retina is a highly specialized, multi-layered sensory tissue which lines the inner surface of the eye, responsible for converting light into electrical neural signals that the brain processes into visual images. Structurally, the retina is composed of multiple layers, each contributing to different aspects of visual processing. The outermost layer, the *retinal pigment epithelium* (RPE), acts as a protective barrier and regulatory interface. It maintains the health of photoreceptors by recycling visual pigments, phagocytosing shed photoreceptor outer segments, and absorbing scattered light, which enhances image clarity and reduces phototoxicity.

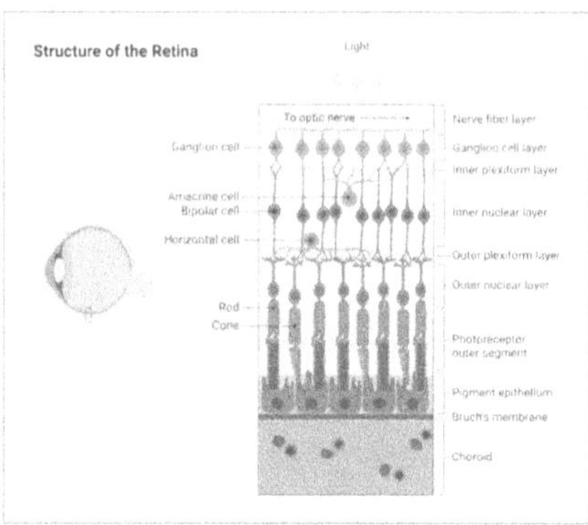

Retinal Layers

Overlying the RPE are *photoreceptors*, which include rods and cones. These cells are responsible for capturing light and initiating the process of phototransduction, converting light energy into electrical energy. Rods, which are highly sensitive to low light levels, enable night vision, whereas cones are responsible for high acuity and color vision. The photoreceptor layer leads into the *outer nuclear layer*, which houses the cell bodies of these photoreceptors.

The *outer plexiform layer* follows, where synaptic connections between photoreceptors, bipolar cells, and horizontal cells occur. This layer is essential for the initial integration of visual signals, allowing the processing of visual information before it is transmitted further through the retina.

Moving more anteriorly within the retina, the *inner nuclear layer* contains the cell bodies of bipolar, horizontal, and amacrine cells. These cells play critical roles in modulating and refining visual signals, ensuring the visual information relayed to the brain is accurate and well-organized. Next is the *inner plexiform layer*, another synaptic zone, where bipolar cells transmit signals to ganglion cells. The *ganglion cell layer* consists of the cell bodies of ganglion cells, which are the final output neurons of the retina.

Finally, the *retinal nerve fiber layer* (RNFL), composed of the axons of ganglion cells, converges to form the optic nerve, which carries visual information to the brain. This intricate layering and organization of the retina enable it to perform the complex task of translating light into the detailed and color-rich visual perceptions that constitute our sense of sight.

Nerve Fiber Layer

The RNFL is of particular importance in glaucoma. It comprises unmyelinated axons of retinal ganglion cells, which converge at the optic disc to form the optic nerve. In glaucoma, *thinning of the RNFL is a hallmark of disease progression* and is closely correlated with the loss of RGCs. The thinning of the RNFL can be detected using imaging modalities such as optical coherence tomography (OCT), which is widely used in clinical practice for the early diagnosis and management of glaucoma.

The loss of RGCs and thinning of the RNFL disrupt transmission of visual signals, leading to visual field defects characteristic of glaucoma. The pattern of RNFL thinning often follows a specific distribution, with the superior and inferior quadrants being more susceptible to early damage.

This distribution corresponds to the characteristic arcuate scotomas observed in the visual fields of many glaucoma patients.

Ganglion Cells

The retinal ganglion cells (RGCs) are the primary cells affected in glaucoma. RGCs are located in the ganglion cell layer of the retina, which is one of the innermost layers. They receive input from bipolar cells and amacrine cells then transmit visual information through their axons, the retinal nerve fiber layer, which converges to form the optic nerve. In a healthy eye, the retina contains approximately 1.2 million RGCs, but their number can vary significantly between individuals. RGCs are required for transmitting visual information from the retina to the brain, making their degeneration a central feature of glaucomatous damage.

RGCs can be classified into different subtypes based on their size, morphology, and function. The most common types include *parasol cells, which form the magnocellular pathway, and midget cells, which form the parvocellular pathway.* Parasol cells are sensitive to motion and are involved in processing low-resolution visual information, while midget cells are responsible for high-resolution vision and color perception. The differential susceptibility of these RGC subtypes to glaucomatous damage remains an area of active research, with evidence suggesting specific subtypes may be more vulnerable than others in early stages of the process.

Vascular Supply

The retina receives its blood supply from two sources: the *central retinal artery*, which supplies the inner retinal layers including the RGCs, and the *choroidal circulation*, which supplies the outer retinal layers including the photoreceptors. The central retinal artery is a branch of the ophthalmic artery, while the choroidal circulation is derived from the posterior ciliary arteries.

Vascular dysregulation and impaired blood flow have been implicated in the pathogenesis of glaucoma, particularly in normal-tension glaucoma (NTG). Reduced perfusion of the optic nerve head and retina may contribute to RGC apoptosis and the progression of glaucomatous damage. Furthermore, autoregulation of retinal blood flow, which ensures a stable blood supply despite fluctuations in systemic blood pressure, may be compromised contributing to ischemic injury and oxidative stress.

Optic Nerve

The optic nerve, cranial nerve II, is the key component of the visual system transmitting information from the retina to the brain. In glaucoma, it is the primary site of damage, with glaucomatous optic neuropathy resulting from the degeneration of RGC axons.

The optic nerve is composed of axons of RGCs, which converge to form the optic disc, also known as the optic nerve head (ONH). The *ONH is "ground zero" in glaucoma*, as it is where the initial signs of glaucomatous damage, such as cupping and thinning of the neuroretinal rim are observed.

The optic nerve consists of approximately 1.2 million axons in a healthy individual, bundled together and surrounded by glial cells, including astrocytes, oligodendrocytes, and microglia.

It can be divided into four segments: the intraocular (optic disc), intraorbital, intracanalicular, and intracranial segments. The intraocular segment is particularly vulnerable to glaucomatous damage, as it is exposed to the biomechanical stress exerted by elevated intraocular pressure (IOP) on the lamina cribrosa - the sieve-like structure through which the RGC axons pass as they exit the eye. Deformation of the lamina cribrosa due to elevated IOP or other factors can lead to mechanical compression and disruption of axonal transport, resulting in RGC death.

Optic Nerve Vascular Supply

The blood supply to the optic nerve is provided by the *short posterior ciliary arteries*, which form a network of capillaries within the optic nerve head. The *central retinal artery* also contributes to the blood supply of the optic disc. In glaucoma, compromised blood flow to the optic nerve head, due to factors such as systemic hypotension or vascular dysregulation, may exacerbate the ischemic damage to RGCs and contribute to the progression of optic neuropathy.

The vascular theory emphasizes the role of impaired blood flow and ischemia in the pathogenesis of glaucomatous optic neuropathy. Reduced perfusion pressure and impaired autoregulation of blood flow to the optic nerve head are thought to contribute to the neuropathy, particularly in patients with normal-tension glaucoma. Understanding the relationship between vascular factors and optic nerve integrity is key for developing and utilizing targeted therapies which address these mechanisms.

Optic Nerve Glial Cells

Glial cells, including astrocytes and microglia, play an essential role in maintaining the integrity of the optic nerve. *Astrocytes* provide structural support and regulate the extracellular environment, while *microglia* act as the resident immune cells, responding to injury and inflammation. In glaucoma, glial cells undergo reactive changes which contribute to the neuroinflammatory processes implicated in RGC death.

Astrocytes in the optic nerve head become activated in response to glaucomatous injury, characterized by hypertrophy and increased expression of glial fibrillary acidic protein (GFAP). These reactive astrocytes may contribute to the remodeling of the extracellular matrix and the formation of glial fibrosis, which can impede axonal regeneration and exacerbate optic nerve damage. Microglia also become activated, releasing pro-inflammatory cytokines and reactive oxygen species that contribute to RGC apoptosis and optic nerve degeneration.

Visual Pathway

The visual pathway is responsible for transmitting visual information from the retina to the brain, where it is processed and interpreted. In glaucoma, damage to RGCs and their axons in the optic nerve leads to a disruption in this pathway, resulting in characteristic visual field defects.

Optic Chiasm & Optic Tracts

The optic nerve from each eye converges at the optic chiasm, located at the base of the brain, where fibers from the nasal half of each retina decussate to the opposite side. This crossing allows visual information from the left visual field of both eyes to be processed in the right hemisphere of the brain, and vice versa. After the chiasm, the fibers continue as the optic tracts, which project to the lateral geniculate nucleus (LGN) of the thalamus.

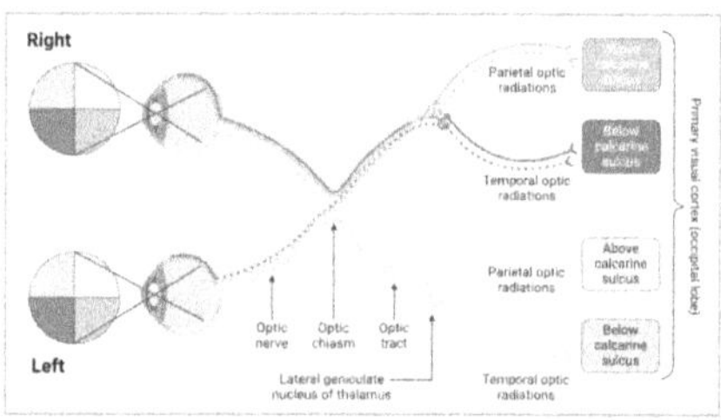

Visual Pathway

Due to its anatomic relationship to the pituitary gland which sits within the sella turcica, the *optic chiasm is a critical site where lesions can cause specific visual field defects*. For example, compression of the optic chiasm by a pituitary adenoma can result in a characteristic bitemporal hemianopic visual field defect. In glaucoma, however, the primary site of damage is the optic nerve, often leading to classic arcuate scotomas and nasal step defects that respect the horizontal midline.

Lateral Geniculate Nucleus

The lateral geniculate nucleus is the *primary relay center for visual information in the thalamus*. It receives input from the optic tracts and sends projections to the primary visual cortex via the optic radiations. The LGN is organized into six layers, with input from the contralateral eye being relayed to layers 1, 4, and 6, and input from the ipsilateral eye being relayed to layers 2, 3, and 5.

In glaucoma, degeneration of RGCs and their axons can lead to retrograde trans-synaptic degeneration of neurons in the LGN. This degeneration is thought to contribute to the reduction in visual acuity and contrast sensitivity observed in many patients. Involvement of the LGN in glaucomatous damage highlights the importance of understanding the entire visual pathway when assessing the impact of the condition.

Optic Radiations

The optic radiations are composed of axons which *originate from neurons in the LGN and project to the primary visual cortex* in the occipital lobe. The optic radiations are divided into two bundles: the upper bundle (Baum's loop), which carries information from the inferior visual field, and the lower bundle (Meyer's loop), which carries information from the superior visual field.

Loss of RGCs and their axons in the optic nerve can also lead to disruptions in the optic radiations, additionally contributing to pathognomonic visual field deficits observed. The corresponding pattern of visual field loss will therefore typically follow the distribution of axonal damage originating in the optic nerve, with the inferior and superior arcuate regions being most affected.

Occipital/Visual Cortex

The occipital cortex, located in the posterior fossa, is responsible for *processing visual information received from the LGN*. The primary visual cortex (V1) is the first cortical area to receive input from the optic radiations and is organized retinotopically, meaning that different regions of the retina correspond to specific areas of V1.

The primary visual cortex is located in the calcarine sulcus of the occipital lobe. It is organized into six layers, with input from the LGN being relayed to layer 4. V1 is responsible for processing basic visual information, such as orientation, contrast, and spatial frequency, which is then relayed to higher visual areas for further processing.

Degeneration of RGCs and their axons in the optic nerve can eventually lead to retrograde degeneration of neurons in V1. This degeneration may ultimately contribute to further reduction in visual acuity and contrast sensitivity observed in these individuals. In addition, loss of input from long-standing glaucomatous optic neuropathy can lead to cortical reorganization, where the representation of the visual field in V1 is altered in response to loss of peripheral vision.

Higher Visual Processing

Beyond V1, visual information is further processed in *several higher cortical areas*, each responsible for different aspects of vision. The dorsal visual stream, also known as the "where" pathway, processes spatial location and movement, while the ventral visual stream, known as the "what" pathway, is involved in object recognition and form representation.

Loss of RGCs and resulting visual field deficits can impact higher visual processing, leading to difficulties with tasks which require spatial awareness, motion detection, and object recognition. Understanding the impact of glaucoma on these higher visual processes is essential for developing and implementing comprehensive rehabilitation strategies for individuals with advanced vision loss.

Chapter 3

Risk Factors & Screening Strategies

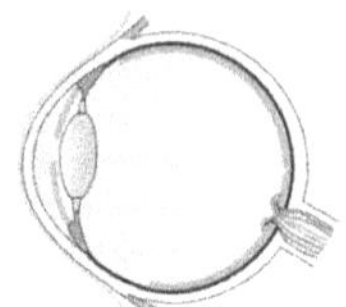

Understanding risk factors in glaucoma is very important for identifying susceptible individuals and implementing early detection strategies. Early detection is essential to prevent or delay the progression of glaucomatous optic neuropathy and loss of vision.

Intraocular Pressure

IOP is the most significant and well-established risk factor in the development of glaucoma. While not all individuals with elevated IOP develop glaucoma, those with *high IOP are at increased risk*. Lowering IOP is known to reduce the risk of progression in both primary open-angle glaucoma and normal-tension glaucoma. However, the relationship between IOP and glaucoma is complex, with some individuals developing significant glaucomatous optic neuropathy at relatively low IOP levels, while others with high IOP may not develop glaucoma at all. This variability underscores the importance of individualized management.

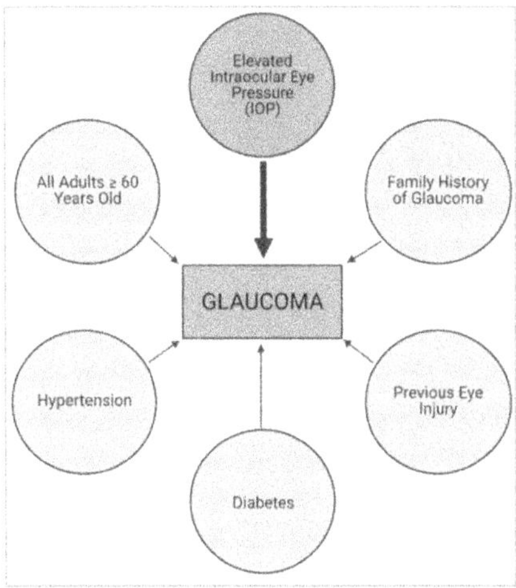

Common Risk Factors in Glaucoma

Age

Age is a major risk factor in glaucoma, with the prevalence of the condition increasing with advancing age. The risk of developing one of the many glaucoma's such as primary open angle glaucoma, narrow angle glaucoma (NAG), or angle closure glaucoma is *significantly increased in individuals over the age of 40*, and the likelihood of glaucoma-related visual impairment rises in older populations as well. Age-related changes in the trabecular meshwork, optic nerve head, and ocular perfusion likely contribute to the increased susceptibility to glaucoma in older individuals. Additionally, older adults may have other comorbidities such as cardiovascular disease or diabetes, which can further increase the risk of glaucoma and complicate its management.

Family History & Genetics

A positive family history of glaucoma is a significant risk factor, suggesting a strong genetic component to the condition. First-degree relatives of individuals with glaucoma have a 4- to 9-fold increased risk of its development. Genetic studies have identified *several loci associated with glaucoma*, including mutations in MYOC, OPTN, and CYP1B1, which contribute to susceptibility in different types of glaucoma. Understanding the genetic basis of glaucoma has important implications for screening and early detection, particularly in families with a known history. Genetic counseling and testing may be appropriate for individuals at high risk allowing for more personalized and proactive management approaches.

Ethnicity

Ethnicity plays a significant role in risk. *African Americans and Hispanics* are at higher risk for primary open-angle glaucoma, with African Americans also experiencing more rapid disease progression and earlier onset. Asian populations are at increased risk for angle-closure glaucoma, particularly those of East Asian descent. The reasons for these ethnic differences in glaucoma risk are multifactorial, involving genetic, anatomical, and environmental factors. For example, African Americans are more likely to have thinner central corneas and larger optic discs which may contribute to their increased susceptibility. In contrast, the shallow anterior chamber depth common in East Asians predisposes them to narrow-angle and angle-closure mechanisms.

Central Corneal Thickness

Central corneal thickness (CCT) is an important factor in assessing the risk of glaucoma, as it can affect the accuracy of IOP measurements, and is also widely accepted as an *independent risk factor*. Thinner corneas are associated with a higher risk of developing glaucoma and are more susceptible to glaucomatous damage. CCT is particularly relevant in individuals with ocular hypertension, where it can help differentiate between those at high risk for progression and those who may be safely monitored without treatment. In addition, CCT can skew the interpretation of IOP readings, as thinner corneas may lead to underestimation and thicker corneas to overestimation of true IOP.

High Myopia

High myopia is a significant risk factor in glaucoma, particularly when the *refractive error exceeds -6.00 diopters*, or the axial length of the eye is greater than 26.5 mm. At these levels, the structural changes induced by axial elongation can lead to thinning and stretching of the sclera, retina, and optic nerve resulting in increased susceptibility to glaucomatous damage. The optic nerve in highly myopic eyes often has features such as a tilted or anomalous anatomic disc (disc-at-risk), peripapillary atrophy, or more pronounced optic nerve cupping. These structural anomalies can also complicate the clinical assessment and may mask or mimic glaucomatous changes making early diagnosis particularly challenging in this population.

Moreover, the mechanical stretching of ocular tissues associated with high myopia exacerbates the vulnerability of retinal ganglion cells to intraocular pressure related stress, even at normal or mildly elevated levels. Consequently, individuals with high myopia are at a significantly greater risk of developing normal-tension glaucoma and may experience more rapid progression. This underscores the importance of vigilant monitoring and tailored management strategies in highly myopic eyes.

Screening Strategies

While *population-based screening for glaucoma remains a topic of debate*, there is evidence to suggest screening older adults and those with known risk factors can be cost-effective and beneficial in reducing the incidence of vision loss due to glaucoma.

High-Risk Populations

Given the asymptomatic nature of early glaucoma, targeted screenings of high-risk populations can be very important for early detection. This includes individuals with *elevated intraocular pressure, a positive family history of glaucoma, African American or Hispanic ethnicity, and older adults*. Regular comprehensive eye exams including IOP measurement, optic nerve head evaluation, and visual fields, are recommended for these groups. Early detection through targeted screening can significantly reduce the risk of vision loss by allowing for timely intervention and management. In addition, education and awareness campaigns aimed at high-risk populations can help increase participation in screening programs and improve adherence to follow-up care.

Technological advancements such as telemedicine and portable diagnostic devices may facilitate broader screening efforts, particularly in underserved areas. Population-based screening programs should be tailored to the specific needs of the population, considering factors such as prevalence, access to care, and availability of resources. For example, in countries with high rates of angle-closure glaucoma, screening programs may focus on identifying individuals with narrow angles or early signs of angle closure. In regions with high rates of open angle glaucoma, screening may prioritize intraocular pressure measurement and optic nerve evaluations.

General Population

For the general population, regarding glaucoma specifically, the American Academy of Ophthalmology (AAO) recommends a *baseline comprehensive eye examination at age 40*, followed by regular exams every 2 to 4 years for individuals aged 40 to 54, every 1 to 3 years for those aged 55 to 64, and every 1 to 2 years for those aged 65 and older. These recommendations are designed to detect early signs of glaucoma, particularly in individuals who may not yet exhibit symptoms. Of course, the timing and frequency of these evaluations may be adjusted based on the presence of risk factors such as elevated intraocular pressure, family history of glaucoma, or other ocular or underlying medical conditions increasing risk.

Pediatrics

Screening for congenital glaucoma is critical for early diagnosis and treatment. Newborns and infants with symptoms such as excessive *tearing, photophobia, or corneal enlargement* should undergo a thorough ophthalmic examination. This includes measurement of IOP, gonioscopy, and optic nerve assessment. Early intervention is imperative in congenital glaucoma to prevent irreversible vision loss. Pediatricians and primary care providers play an essential role in identifying at-risk infants and referring them for specialized care. For children with a family history of congenital glaucoma or other risk factors, regular monitoring and early screening are recommended even in the absence of symptoms.

The Underserved

Underserved populations, including those in *rural areas or with limited access to healthcare*, may benefit from targeted screening programs that utilize portable diagnostic devices, telemedicine, and community-based initiatives. These efforts can help identify at-risk individuals or those with glaucoma who may not otherwise have access to regular eye care, reducing the burden of the condition in these populations. Partnerships with local healthcare providers, community organizations, and government agencies can help expand access to screening and treatment services ensuring even the most vulnerable populations are addressed.

Chapter 4
The Glaucoma's

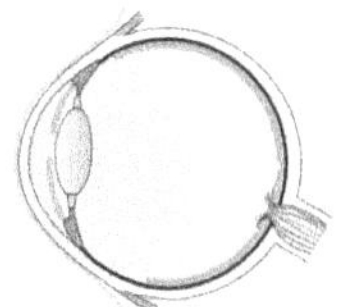

Glaucoma represents a diverse group of optic neuropathies characterized by the *progressive degeneration of retinal ganglion cells*, leading to structural damage to the optic nerve and subsequent visual field loss. The disease can manifest with decreased visual acuity and contrast sensitivity, particularly as it advances. While elevated intraocular pressure has long been identified as a significant risk factor, it is now recognized that glaucoma is a multifactorial disease. Various subtypes exist, each with distinct pathophysiological mechanisms, clinical presentations, and management strategies. These subtypes include Primary Open-Angle Glaucoma, Angle-Closure Glaucoma, Normal-Tension Glaucoma, Secondary Glaucoma, and Congenital Glaucoma.

The complex pathophysiology of glaucoma has led to an evolution in its definition by leading professional bodies such as the American Optometric Association (AOA) and the American Academy of Ophthalmology (AAO). These organizations have *de-emphasized the role of intraocular pressure* as the sole defining feature of glaucoma. Instead, glaucoma is now more accurately described as a group of eye disorders characterized by progressive optic nerve damage, which, if left untreated, can result in irreversible vision loss. This shift in definition acknowledges the diversity in the mechanisms of optic nerve damage, which extends beyond mere IOP elevation.

The AAO describes glaucoma as a condition often associated with elevated IOP, but it is the optic nerve damage that serves as the hallmark of the disease. This damage results from a combination of mechanical stress and vascular factors, leading to the characteristic pattern of vision loss seen in glaucoma patients. On the other hand, the AOA emphasizes the critical importance of early detection through comprehensive eye examinations. This approach is particularly pertinent in cases of normal-tension glaucoma, where optic nerve damage occurs even in the absence of elevated IOP. The AOA highlights the need for thorough optic nerve head assessments and functional testing, including optical coherence tomography and visual field analysis, to identify glaucomatous changes early, even when IOP levels are within the normal range.

Primary Open-Angle

Primary open angle glaucoma (POAG) is the most common form of glaucoma, accounting for approximately 74% of all cases worldwide. This condition is characterized by an open anterior chamber angle and a progressive increase in IOP due to impaired drainage of aqueous humor through the trabecular meshwork. The defining feature of POAG is an *open angle between the cornea and the iris which is not obstructed*, however, the drainage system becomes inefficient over time. Its pathophysiology involves a gradual increase in resistance to aqueous humor outflow within the trabecular meshwork, which may be due to several factors, including abnormal extracellular matrix deposition, endothelial dysfunction, or alterations in the cytoskeleton of trabecular cells. These changes result in elevated IOP, which exerts mechanical stress on the optic nerve head, particularly at the level of the lamina cribrosa, leading to axonal damage and RGC death.

Its course is typically chronic and progressive, with the rate of progression varying among individuals. Genetic factors play a significant role in susceptibility, with *mutations in genes such as MYOC (myocilin), OPTN (optineurin), and CYP1B1* being associated with an increased risk of developing the condition. The identification of these genetic factors has enhanced our understanding of the heritability of POAG and has opened avenues for potential gene-targeted therapies in the future.

Clinically, POAG is often asymptomatic in its early stages, leading to its description as the "silent thief of sight." This lack of symptoms poses a significant challenge for early detection, as individuals typically do not notice visual changes until the disease has progressed substantially. When symptoms do appear, they often manifest as visual field defects that progress slowly over time, usually beginning with peripheral field loss. Central vision remains intact until the disease reaches an advanced stage, making early detection crucial to preventing irreversible vision loss.

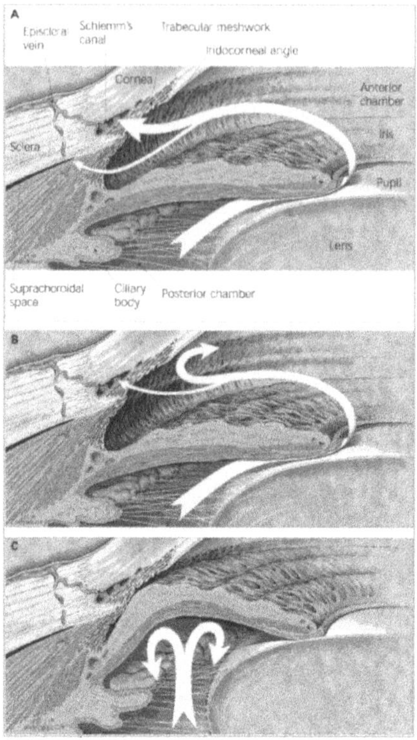

Anterior Chamber Aqueous Flow

Diagnosis of POAG relies on a combination of clinical findings. While elevated IOP is a common feature, it is not always present, as POAG can also occur at normal IOP levels. Key diagnostic indicators include characteristic optic nerve head changes, such as an increased cup-to-disc ratio and thinning of the neuroretinal rim, as well as visual field defects detected using standard automated perimetry. Imaging modalities such as optical coherence tomography have become the standard of care, allowing for the assessment of retinal nerve fiber layer thickness and the detection of early glaucomatous changes that may not be apparent on clinical examination alone.

The primary goal of POAG management is to lower IOP to a level that prevents further optic neuropathy and preserves visual function. This can be achieved through various approaches, including *pharmacological treatments, laser therapy, and surgical interventions*. First-line pharmacological treatments typically include prostaglandin analogs, beta-blockers, alpha agonists, and carbonic anhydrase inhibitors, which work by either reducing aqueous humor production or increasing its outflow. For patients who do not respond adequately to medical treatment, laser trabeculoplasty, particularly selective laser trabeculoplasty (SLT), offers an effective alternative. In more advanced cases, or when pharmacological and laser treatments fail, surgical procedures such as trabeculectomy or glaucoma drainage device implantation may be necessary to achieve adequate IOP control.

Narrow Angle

Narrow angle glaucoma (NAG) is characterized by an anatomically reduced anterior chamber angle, where the *space between the iris and the trabecular meshwork is significantly diminished*. This anatomical narrowing predisposes the eye to potential blockage of aqueous outflow, leading to increased intraocular pressure and a heightened risk of developing angle closure glaucoma. It often remains asymptomatic until the angle becomes critically narrow, at which point it can cause intermittent or sustained elevations in IOP.

Narrowing of the anterior chamber angle can be influenced by several factors including the *natural aging process, hyperopia, as well as anatomic variations such as a shallow anterior chamber or bulky lens.* Under normal conditions, aqueous produced by the ciliary body flows through the pupil into the anterior chamber and exits via the trabecular meshwork. In eyes with narrow angles, this outflow pathway is compromised due to reduced angle width, particularly during pupillary dilation or mydriasis. Situations which induce mydriasis, such as low light conditions, stress, or the use of certain pharmacological agents (e.g., anticholinergics, adrenergics) can exacerbate the narrowing. This further obstructs aqueous outflow leading to transient or sustained IOP elevation with angle closure, especially if left unmonitored or untreated. An acute episode of angle closure can occur if the anterior chamber angle closes abruptly, leading to rapid, painful, and severe increase in IOP which can induce immediate glaucomatous neuropathy and vision loss if not promptly treated.

To prevent the progression from narrow angle glaucoma to angle closure glaucoma, regular monitoring is key. This involves periodic gonioscopy to assess the angle's width and structure, as well as IOP measurements and optic nerve evaluations. Prophylactic treatment is often recommended for individuals at high risk of angle closure. *Laser peripheral iridotomy* (LPI) is the most common prophylactic procedure, in which a small opening is created in the peripheral iris using a laser. This opening allows aqueous to bypass the narrow pupillary pathway and flow directly into the anterior chamber, reducing risk of angle closure by flattening the iris and widening the angle.

Narrow angle glaucoma represents a critical anatomic stage requiring vigilant observation and timely intervention to prevent acute or chronic angle closure, and thus preserve optic nerve function.

Angle-Closure

Angle-closure glaucoma (ACG) is another major subtype of glaucoma. ACG is characterized by the *closure of the anterior chamber angle*, which obstructs the outflow of aqueous humor and leads to elevated IOP. Although ACG is less common than POAG, it tends to be more severe and can result in rapid vision loss if not promptly treated. The pathophysiology of ACG involves anatomical predispositions such as a shallow anterior chamber, a thickened lens, or a combination of both. These anatomical features increase the risk of angle closure, which can occur through various mechanisms, including pupillary block, plateau iris configuration, or lens-induced factors such as phacomorphic glaucoma.

Pupillary block is the most common mechanism of angle closure. It occurs when the lens blocks the flow of aqueous humor from the posterior chamber to the anterior chamber, leading to a forward bowing of the iris and subsequent angle closure. Plateau iris configuration, on the other hand, occurs when the peripheral iris is pushed forward due to an abnormal insertion of the ciliary body, even in the absence of a pupillary block. In addition, lens-induced angle closure can occur in cases of lens subluxation or anterior lens displacement, as seen in hypermature cataracts.

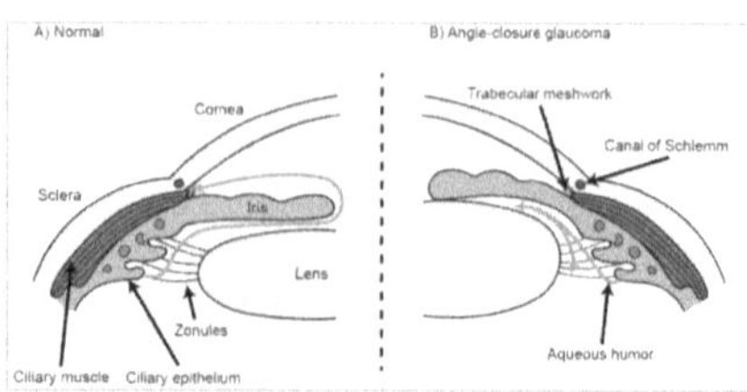

Open vs Closed Angle

ACG can present in various clinical forms, ranging from acute to chronic. Acute angle-closure glaucoma (AACG) is a true ophthalmic emergency characterized by the sudden onset of severe ocular pain, headache, decreased vision, halos around lights, and nausea or vomiting. The affected eye typically shows intense episcleral and conjunctival injection, a mid-dilated non-reactive or sluggish pupil, and corneal haze secondary to corneal edema. IOP is markedly elevated often exceeding 40-50 mmHg. If untreated, AACG can lead to permanent vision loss within hours to days. Chronic angle-closure glaucoma (CACG), on the other hand, progresses more slowly and may be asymptomatic until significant optic nerve damage has occurred. CACG may present with episodes of subacute angle closure which cause transient symptoms of mild pain and blurred vision, often occurring in low-light conditions where the pupil dilates.

The management of ACG differs from that of POAG due to its urgency. In acute cases, *immediate intervention is required to lower IOP* and prevent permanent glaucomatous optic neuropathy. Initial treatment typically includes medications such as oral carbonic anhydrase inhibitors, oral hyperosmotic agents (e.g., mannitol), and topical beta-blockers or alpha agonists to reduce IOP. *Emergent Nd:YAG laser peripheral iridotomy* is the key treatment for pupillary block ACG, creating an opening in the peripheral iris to allow aqueous humor to bypass the block and enter the anterior chamber. In cases where LPI is insufficient, additional procedures such as laser iridoplasty, lens extraction, or glaucoma filtration surgery may be necessary.

Normal-Tension

Normal tension glaucoma (NTG) was previously described as low-tension glaucoma, and is a subtype of POAG in which *optic neuropathy and visual field loss occur despite normal IOP* levels. NTG presents a significant diagnostic and therapeutic challenge, as the pathophysiological mechanisms are not fully understood and differ from those in POAG with elevated IOP. The exact pathophysiology of NTG remains unclear, but several factors are thought to contribute to optic neuropathy in the absence of elevated IOP.

Vascular dysregulation is a key hypothesis in NTG, where impaired blood flow and autoregulation to the optic nerve lead to inadequate perfusion and ischemic injury. Systemic factors such as nocturnal hypotension, vasospastic disorders, and cardiovascular disease may exacerbate this vascular insufficiency. Another proposed mechanism involves increased susceptibility of the optic nerve head to biomechanical stress, even at normal IOP levels. Structural factors, such as a thinner and more fragile lamina cribrosa or greater physiological optic disc cupping, may predispose the optic nerve to glaucomatous damage under lower IOP conditions.

NTG presents clinically in a manner similar to POAG, with progressive visual field loss and characteristic glaucomatous optic neuropathy, but without elevated IOP. Interestingly, individuals with NTG often have more pronounced visual field defects that are closer to fixation compared to those with "high-tension" POAG. Additionally, NTG is more commonly associated with splinter hemorrhages at the optic disc margin, a finding that may indicate progressive optic neuropathy.

The diagnosis of NTG requires careful assessment to *rule out secondary causes of optic neuropathy*, such as ischemic optic neuropathy, compressive lesions, or optic neuritis. Detailed history-taking, including an assessment of vascular risk factors, blood pressure management (particularly nocturnal hypotension), and neuroimaging may be necessary. Despite its normal baseline IOP levels, the management of NTG still focuses on lowering IOP, as studies have shown reducing IOP in NTG can slow the progression of optic neuropathy. Treatment options are similar to those for POAG, including *topical medications, laser therapy, and surgery*. However, the target IOP is typically set much lower for NTG patients, often aiming for a reduction of at least 30% or more from baseline. Non-IOP lowering strategies must also be considered, particularly in patients with evidence of vascular dysregulation. These strategies include optimizing systemic blood pressure, particularly at night, and *addressing cardiovascular risk factors*. Neuroprotective agents such as calcium channel blockers have recently been explored in NTG, but their efficacy remains uncertain.

Secondary Glaucoma's

This refers to a group of glaucoma's where elevated IOP and optic nerve damage are secondary to an identifiable underlying etiology. These scenarios can be broadly classified into open-angle and angle-closure mechanisms.

Pigmentary

Pigmentary glaucoma (PG) is an open-angle secondary glaucoma caused by the *dispersion of iris pigment granules into the anterior chamber*. These pigment granules accumulate in the trabecular meshwork, leading to increased outflow resistance and elevated IOP. The condition is often seen in young, myopic individuals and is also known as pigment dispersion syndrome. Clinically, pigmentary glaucoma presents with symptoms such as intermittent blurring of vision, halos around lights, and elevated IOP, particularly after activities that increase pigment release, such as vigorous exercise or eye rubbing. The management of pigmentary glaucoma typically involves IOP-lowering therapies similar to those used in POAG, with a focus on maintaining open-angle trabecular function.

Pseudoexfoliative

Pseudoexfoliative glaucoma (PXG) is another form of secondary open-angle glaucoma, occurring in association with pseudoexfoliation syndrome (PXS). PXS is an age-related systemic condition characterized by the *production and accumulation of abnormal fibrillar extracellular material* on various ocular structures, including the lens, iris, and trabecular meshwork. This material obstructs aqueous humor outflow, leading to elevated IOP. PXG is more common in older adults and has been linked with systemic vascular disease. Clinically, PXG can be more aggressive than POAG, with higher IOP levels, greater fluctuations in IOP, and a higher risk of optic nerve damage. Management of PXG involves aggressive IOP control, often requiring a combination of pharmacological, laser, and surgical treatments.

Neovascular

Neovascular glaucoma (NVG) is an angle-closure secondary glaucoma created by the growth and proliferation of abnormal new blood vessels, *neovascularization, in the anterior chamber angle*. It is often secondary to ischemic retinal conditions, such as advanced proliferative diabetic retinopathy or central retinal vein occlusion. The abnormal neovascular vessels obstruct aqueous outflow, leading to a rapid increase in IOP. Neovascular glaucoma is challenging to manage and requires aggressive medical and surgical intervention. Pan-retinal photocoagulation (PRP) laser treatment and/or intravitreal anti-VEGF therapy are often employed to reduce neovascularization and control IOP. In more advanced cases, surgical options such as glaucoma drainage device implantation may be necessary.

Uveitic

Uveitic glaucoma (UG) is a form of secondary glaucoma which develops in conjunction with uveitis, an inflammation of the uveal tract, which includes the iris, ciliary body, and choroid.

This inflammation can lead to an increase in IOP through various mechanisms. One of the primary causes is the *obstruction of the trabecular meshwork by inflammatory cells, debris, and proteins* accumulating in the anterior chamber, which impedes aqueous humor outflow and results in elevated IOP. Treatment of uveitis often involves the use of corticosteroids, which, while effective in reducing inflammation, can induce an increase in IOP in some individuals, further complicating management. Chronic inflammation may also lead to the formation of synechiae, which are adhesions between the iris and lens (posterior synechiae) or between the iris and cornea (anterior synechiae). These adhesions can contribute to the development of angle-closure glaucoma via pupillary block or obstruction of the trabecular meshwork. Managing uveitic glaucoma is particularly challenging because it requires *simultaneous control of both the underlying uveitis and the elevated IOP*. Treatment typically involves a combination of anti-inflammatory medications to address the uveitis, IOP-lowering therapies, and addressing the underlying etiology, such as in cases of rheumatologic conditions and autoimmunity.

Congenital Glaucoma

This is also known as primary congenital glaucoma (PCG), a rare but severe form of glaucoma presenting in infancy or early childhood. It is caused by *developmental abnormalities in the anterior chamber angle* obstructing aqueous outflow. The pathophysiology of congenital glaucoma involves maldevelopment of the trabecular meshwork and Schlemm's canal, and may be due to genetic mutations with CYP1B1 being the most implicated gene. Elevated IOP in congenital glaucoma can lead to increasing axial length and physical enlargement of the eye (buphthalmos), corneal edema, and subsequent optic neuropathy or atrophy.

Clinically, congenital glaucoma typically presents with a classic triad of symptoms: *epiphora, blepharospasm, and photophobia*. On examination, the eye is often noticeably enlarged, and the cornea may appear hazy due to associated stromal edema. Evidence of corneal enlargement or megalocornea is usually apparent. Diagnosis is confirmed through clinical examination, including measurement of IOP, assessment of the anterior chamber angle using gonioscopy, and evaluation of the optic nerve for signs of glaucomatous damage. Ultrasound can also support the diagnosis, providing information on anterior chamber anatomy and overall axial length.

The *management of congenital glaucoma is primarily surgical*, as medical therapy alone is often insufficient to control IOP in these individuals. Goniotomy or trabeculotomy are the procedures of choice, aimed at opening the trabecular meshwork to allow for improved aqueous outflow. In cases where these procedures are unsuccessful, trabeculectomy or glaucoma drainage device implantation may be required. Early diagnosis and intervention are critical in congenital glaucoma to prevent irreversible optic atrophy and severe vision loss. Long-term follow-up is essential, as these patients are at risk for chronic ocular hypertension with progressive glaucomatous optic neuropathy throughout their lives.

Chapter 5

Pathophysiology

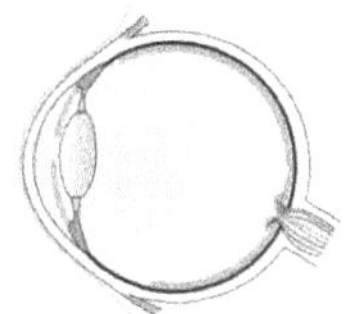

Multifactorial Pathophysiology

The pathophysiology of glaucoma is complex and involves a multifactorial interplay of *genetic, environmental, and biological factors*. Central to the disease process is the progressive loss of RGCs, which results in optic nerve damage and subsequent visual field loss. However, the mechanisms underlying RGC death and optic nerve degeneration are not fully understood and likely vary among different forms of glaucoma.

Biomechanical Factors & Vascular Theory of Glaucoma

The relationship between IOP and mechanically induced glaucomatous optic neuropathy is not straightforward. For example, some individuals with high IOP do not develop glaucoma but instead purely ocular hypertension (OHTN), while others progress despite lowering IOP. The Ocular

Hypertension Treatment Study (OHTS) reported that over *90% of individuals with high IOP did not progress to glaucoma over a five-year period*, suggesting factors beyond IOP contribute to the disease process.

Biomechanical factors

These are physical contributors in the pathogenesis of glaucoma, particularly through their influence on the optic nerve head and lamina cribrosa (LC). The LC is a specialized structure within the ONH, composed of collagenous beams forming a meshwork through which RGC axons pass as they exit the eye. IOP exerts a *mechanical load on the LC*, leading to its deformation, posterior displacement, and thickening. These biomechanical changes disrupt axonal transport within the RGCs, leading to their progressive degeneration and death, ultimately resulting in glaucomatous optic neuropathy.

The susceptibility of the ONH to biomechanical stress is influenced by several factors, including the composition and geometry of the LC, the connective tissue surrounding it, and the overall structural integrity of the optic nerve. Individuals with a thinner or more compliant LC may be more vulnerable to IOP-induced damage, even at relatively normal IOP levels, as seen in cases of normal-tension glaucoma. Additionally, age-related changes in the sclera, such as decreased collagen cross-linking, can alter its biomechanical properties, leading to increased strain on the ONH and LC. These alterations may exacerbate the mechanical vulnerability of the optic nerve, further contributing to the development and progression of glaucoma. The interplay between these biomechanical factors underscores the complexity of glaucoma pathophysiology and highlights the need for therapeutic approaches that target not only IOP reduction but also the structural integrity and biomechanical environment of the ONH.

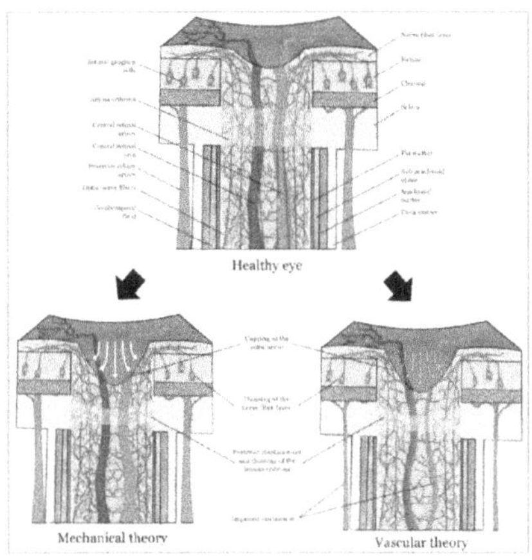

Mechanical vs Vascular Theory

Vascular

The vascular theory supports that compromised ocular blood flow plays a key role in the pathogenesis of glaucomatous optic neuropathy. Reduced ocular blood flow and unstable oxygen supply have been reported in various vascular beds of glaucoma patients. According to this theory, insufficient perfusion of the optic nerve head due to vascular dysregulation, impaired autoregulation, or systemic vascular conditions leads to ischemia and subsequent retinal ganglion cell death. The ONH, being highly metabolically active, is particularly vulnerable to fluctuations in blood supply. Reduced ocular perfusion pressure (OPP), defined as the difference between blood pressure and intraocular pressure, has been strongly associated with the risk of glaucoma development and progression. Low OPP may result from either elevated IOP, systemic hypotension, or a combination of both leading to a delicate balance where even mild reductions in blood flow can precipitate ischemic injury to the optic nerve.

One of the key aspects of the vascular theory is the *role of autoregulation*, the process by which blood vessels maintain constant blood flow despite changes in perfusion pressure. In healthy individuals, autoregulation ensures the optic nerve head receives an adequate blood supply even under varying systemic blood pressure. However, in glaucoma patients, particularly those with normal-tension glaucoma, this autoregulatory mechanism may be impaired. Specifically, neurovascular coupling, the process by which neuronal activity regulates blood flow to match metabolic demand is thought to be disrupted. Impaired neurovascular coupling can result in inadequate blood supply especially during periods of increased metabolic activity, exacerbating ischemic damage to the optic nerve. It can also be exacerbated by systemic vascular conditions such as nocturnal hypotension, vasospastic disorders, and vascular endothelial dysfunction, only further compromising blood supply to the ONH. In terms of vascular endothelial dysfunction, once perfusion pressure declines beyond a critical range, vascular endothelial autoregulation begins to break down. This is characterized by an imbalance between vasodilators (e.g., nitric oxide) and vasoconstrictors (e.g., endothelin-1). In general, if for any reason autoregulation fails, the resulting hypoxia and oxidative stress within the optic nerve head creates an environment conducive to RGC apoptosis, thus contributing to the progression of glaucomatous damage.

Several vascular factors play a critical role in the pathophysiology, influencing both intraocular pressure dynamics and optic nerve integrity. Among these factors, nitric oxide (NO), endothelin-1 (ET-1), and vascular endothelial growth factor (VEGF) are of particular importance due to their impact on ocular blood flow and vascular regulation.

- **Nitric oxide** is a key molecule involved in the regulation of vasodilation within the eye. It facilitates the relaxation of blood vessels, thereby promoting adequate blood flow to the optic nerve and other ocular structures. In glaucoma patients, reduced levels of nitric oxide are associated with decreased vasodilation and increased vasoconstriction, which can compromise optic nerve perfusion and exacerbate glaucomatous damage. The diminished availability of NO may contribute to the vascular dysregulation often observed in glaucoma, particularly in forms such as normal-tension glaucoma.

- **Endothelin-1** is a potent vasoconstrictor, and its role in glaucoma has been increasingly recognized. Elevated levels of endothelin-1 have been detected in both the plasma and aqueous humor of glaucoma patients. This elevation is believed to contribute to the pathological vasoconstriction seen in glaucoma, reducing blood flow to the optic nerve head and potentially leading to ischemic damage. The heightened presence of endothelin-1 may also interact with other factors to exacerbate the progression of glaucomatous optic neuropathy.

- **Vascular endothelial growth factor** is another critical factor, particularly in the context of ocular hypoxia. VEGF is upregulated in hypoxic environments, such as those found in the eyes of individuals with glaucoma. Elevated levels of VEGF in the aqueous humor are commonly observed in these patients. While VEGF plays a protective role by promoting angiogenesis in response to hypoxia, its overexpression can lead to pathological changes, including neovascularization, which can further complicate glaucoma management by contributing to secondary forms of the condition, such as neovascular glaucoma.

The vascular theory highlights the importance of considering not only IOP but also the broader cardiovascular status of the entire patient when managing glaucoma. This supports the potential for therapeutic approaches targeting vascular function and perfusion in addition to traditional IOP-lowering strategies.

Neuroinflammatory

The neuroinflammatory theory of glaucoma suggests chronic inflammation within the optic nerve head and retina plays a pivotal role in the pathogenesis of glaucomatous optic neuropathy. This theory supports glaucomatous damage is not solely a consequence of mechanical stress or vascular insufficiency but also involves an active pathological response of the immune system, particularly the innate immune components within the central nervous system.

Key players in this neuroinflammatory process include glial cells, astrocytes, microglia, and Müller cells, which become activated in response to various stressors including elevated intraocular pressure, ischemia, and oxidative stress. Upon activation, these *glial cells release pro-inflammatory cytokines, chemokines, and other neurotoxic factors* which contribute to the progressive degeneration of retinal ganglion cells. These responses occur at early stages in the disease process, with inhibition of certain pro-inflammatory pathways also appearing as a neuroprotective response.

- **Astrocytes**, the most abundant glial cells in the optic nerve head, undergo a process known as reactive gliosis in response to glaucomatous injury. This involves morphological changes, such as hypertrophy and up-regulation of glial fibrillary acidic protein (GFAP), along with the production of inflammatory mediators. While initially protective, chronic astrocyte activity can lead to a harmful environment characterized by increased extracellular matrix deposition and the release of factors which exacerbate axonal damage.

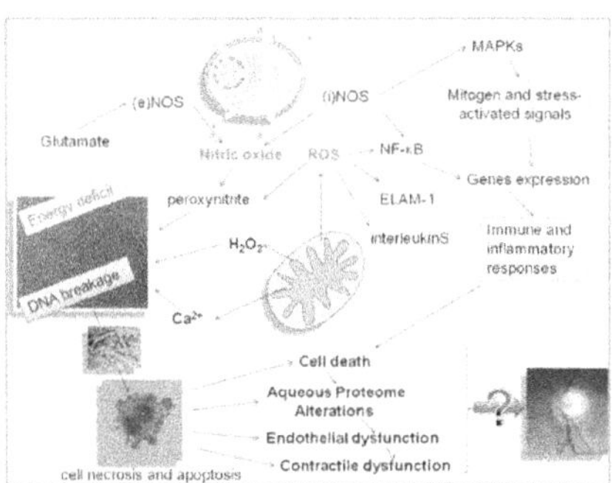

Glaucomatous Neuroinflammation

- **Microglia**, the resident immune cells of the central nervous system, also play a critical role in the neuroinflammatory response. In glaucoma, microglia become activated and migrate to sites of injury where they release pro-inflammatory cytokines like TNF-α, IL-1β, and IL-6, as well as reactive oxygen species (ROS). Fas ligand, a proapoptotic protein, is also implicated in glaucoma pathogenesis through various inflammatory pathways. These factors contribute to the apoptotic pathways leading to RGC death. Additionally, the complement cascade, part of the innate immune system, is up-regulated in glaucoma and has been implicated in synaptic pruning and direct neurodegeneration.

The neuroinflammatory theory provides a framework for understanding glaucoma as a neurodegenerative disease driven by chronic localized inflammation, suggesting therapeutic strategies aimed at modulating glial cell activity and dampening neuroinflammation could be effective in slowing or halting progression.

Genetic & Molecular Basis

The genetic and molecular basis of glaucoma is complex, involving multiple genes and signaling pathways which contribute to the development and progression of this multifactorial condition. Glaucoma is not a single-gene disorder but rather a *polygenic condition* with both Mendelian and non-Mendelian inheritance patterns. Mutations in several genes have been identified in various forms of glaucoma, with the most well-characterized being MYOC, OPTN, and CYP1B1.

These genetic alterations can influence susceptibility to elevated intraocular pressure, optic nerve vulnerability, and overall resilience of retinal ganglion cells to stress and injury.

- **MYOC** (Myocilin) is the gene most associated with primary open-angle glaucoma, particularly in juvenile-onset cases. MYOC mutations can lead to the accumulation of misfolded myocilin proteins in the trabecular meshwork, disrupting normal aqueous humor outflow and resulting in elevated IOP. This increased pressure exerts mechanical stress on the optic nerve head, leading to axonal damage and subsequent RGC death. Interestingly, the exact pathogenic mechanism by which mutant myocilin induces increased IOP and glaucoma remains under investigation, with current research suggesting a role for endoplasmic reticulum stress and activation of apoptotic pathways in trabecular meshwork cells.

- **OPTN** (Optineurin) and TBK1 (TANK-binding kinase 1) mutations are associated with normal-tension glaucoma, where optic nerve damage occurs despite normal IOP levels. OPTN mutations are thought to affect autophagy and neuroprotective mechanisms in RGCs, making them more susceptible to apoptosis. Similarly, TBK1 mutations lead to dysregulation of autophagy, contributing to the accumulation of damaged proteins and organelles ultimately promoting RGC degeneration.

- **CYP1B1** mutations are linked to primary congenital glaucoma, where defective metabolism of signaling molecules such as retinoic acid impairs normal eye development leading to trabecular meshwork malformation and elevated IOP from birth.

Beyond these well-characterized genes, genome-wide association studies (GWAS) have identified numerous single nucleotide polymorphisms (SNPs) in loci related to extracellular matrix remodeling, vascular regulation, and neuroinflammation. For example, SNPs in the CDKN2B-AS1 locus which regulates cell cycle progression and apoptosis have been linked to an increased risk of POAG. Similarly, variants in genes involved in TGF-β signaling, such as TGFBR3, are associated with structural changes in the optic nerve head that predispose individuals to glaucoma. The identification of these genetic factors underscores the complexity of glaucoma's molecular landscape, suggesting the disease arises from a confluence of genetic predisposition, environmental influences, and stochastic events that together compromise optic nerve integrity.

These insights into the genetic and molecular basis of glaucoma have significant implications for the future of diagnosis and treatment. Genetic screening for at-risk individuals, particularly those with a family history of glaucoma, may allow for earlier detection and more personalized therapeutic interventions. Furthermore, understanding the molecular pathways involved in glaucoma pathogenesis opens the door to the development of targeted therapies aimed at modulating specific genetic or molecular defects, potentially altering the disease course and preserving vision in affected individuals.

Chapter 6

Diagnostics & Biomarkers

The diagnosis of glaucoma involves a multifaceted approach, utilizing a combination of clinical examination, imaging techniques, and functional assessments to evaluate the optic nerve head, intraocular pressure, and visual fields.

Tonometry

Tonometry is the diagnostic procedure used to measure intraocular pressure, a key factor in the assessment and management of glaucoma. Elevated IOP is a significant risk factor for glaucoma, making accurate measurement essential for early detection, managing progression, and guiding treatment strategies. Tonometry techniques have evolved significantly over time, with advancements in technology improving the precision, safety, and comfort of IOP measurements.

The origins of tonometry date back to the 19th century, when it was recognized the importance of intraocular pressure in the pathophysiology of glaucoma. One of the pioneering instruments was the Schiøtz tonometer, introduced by Norwegian ophthalmologist Hjalmar Schiøtz in 1905. This indentation tonometer measured IOP by determining the degree of indentation made by a known weight placed on the cornea. Although groundbreaking at the time, the Schiøtz tonometer had limitations, including variability due to corneal properties and the need for patient cooperation.

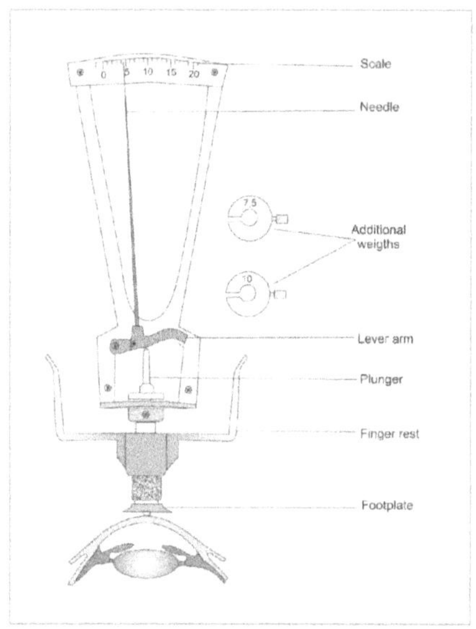

Schiøtz Tonometer

In the mid-20th century, applanation tonometry emerged as the gold standard for IOP measurement, largely due to the work of Hans Goldmann. The *Goldmann applanation tonometer* (GAT), developed in 1957, measures IOP based on the Imbert-Fick principle, which states that the pressure inside a perfectly elastic, dry sphere is equal to the force needed to flatten its surface. By applanating or flattening a small precise area of the cornea, GAT provides an accurate estimation of IOP. This technique remains widely used today and is considered the reference standard against which other tonometers are calibrated.

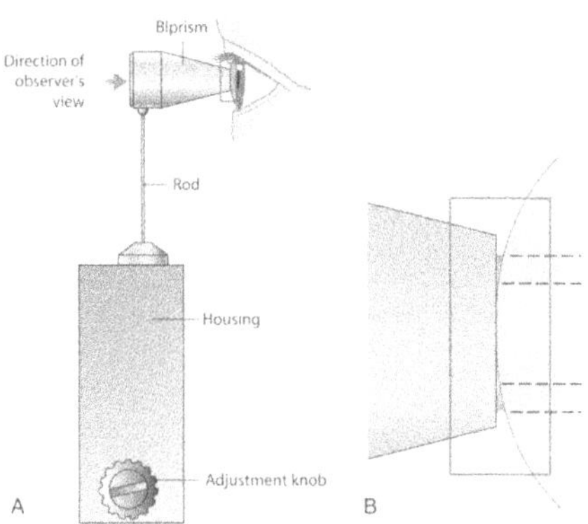

Goldmann Tonometer

Several types of tonometers are currently available, each with specific advantages and limitations. In addition to the Goldmann applanation tonometer, non-contact tonometers (NCT) also known as *"air-puff" tonometers* are commonly used, especially in clinical settings where rapid non-invasive measurements are preferred. NCT works by directing a brief pulse of air at the cornea, flattening it momentarily, and measuring the time taken to achieve this deformation. Although NCT is convenient and eliminates the need for topical anesthesia, it is generally considered less accurate than Goldmann applanation tonometry particularly at higher IOP levels.

The *Perkins tonometer* is a portable handheld version of the Goldmann tonometer, designed for use in situations where a standard slit-lamp-mounted Goldmann tonometer is impractical such as in pediatric or bedridden patients. The

Perkins tonometer offers the same level of accuracy as the Goldmann tonometer making it a valuable tool in various clinical settings.

Another widely used device is the *Tono-Pen*, a handheld applanation tonometer which offers portability and ease of use, making it ideal for use in various clinical environments, including emergency rooms and in hospital settings. The Tono-Pen measures IOP by applying gentle pressure to the cornea incorporating microprocessor technology to average multiple readings improving accuracy.

The *iCare tonometer* is also very popular today. It is a portable handheld device which measures intraocular pressure without the need for anesthesia or corneal contact using a light disposable probe that gently rebounds off the cornea. It is particularly useful for quick patient-friendly assessments in both clinical settings and even at home, making it ideal for individuals who require frequent monitoring. It calculates intraocular pressure by measuring the deceleration of a small lightweight probe as it gently rebounds off the cornea. The device uses the probe's rebound characteristics, specifically the speed and force at which it returns after contacting the cornea, to estimate pressure. The device's microprocessor then analyzes these rebound measurements correlating them with IOP values based on pre-calibrated data, providing an accurate and reliable result.

Dynamic contour tonometry (DCT), such as the Pascal tonometer, represents a more recent advancement in IOP measurement. Unlike applanation methods, DCT measures IOP based on the principle of contour matching which reduces the influence of corneal properties on IOP readings.

This method is particularly advantageous in patients with irregular corneas or after refractive surgery where traditional applanation techniques may be less accurate.

Looking ahead, the future of tonometry is likely to be shaped by the development of devices which offer continuous IOP monitoring as opposed to single point-in-time measurements. Implantable IOP sensors, such as those being developed by companies like Sensimed and Implandata, have the potential to provide real-time 24/7/365 IOP monitoring offering unprecedented insights into pressure variation and its impact on glaucoma progression. These sensors can be integrated into contact lenses or implanted during cataract or glaucoma surgery, enabling seamless and continuous monitoring without the need for repeated office visits.

Smartphone-based tonometry is another area of innovation, with the development of devices which can be attached to smartphones to measure IOP. These devices aim to make measurements more accessible, especially in resource-limited settings by leveraging the widespread availability of smartphones.

Gonioscopy

Gonioscopy is a technique utilized to visualize anterior chamber angle structures and to assess the trabecular meshwork. It is essential in *differentiating between open-angle, narrow-angle, and angle-closure* glaucoma, or identifying potential abnormalities which could impede outflow of aqueous humor leading to elevated intraocular pressure. It provides valuable information that cannot be obtained through routine slit-lamp exams, making it indispensable in comprehensive glaucoma evaluations. It is also necessary when determining treatment strategies, for example, choosing between SLT in an open angle or LPI in a narrow or closed angle.

The origins of gonioscopy can be traced back to the early 20th century. The procedure was first introduced by the Swiss ophthalmologist Alexios Trantas in 1907, who used a direct ophthalmoscope to observe the anterior chamber angle. However, the technique was significantly refined by the Austrian ophthalmologist Maximilian Salzmann, who in 1914 developed a method to visualize the angle using a specialized contact lens. This early iteration of gonioscopy provided a direct view of angle structures, but it was cumbersome and had limitations in terms of image clarity and ease of use.

A major advancement came in 1938 when Thorpe and Barkan introduced the goniolens, a mirrored contact lens which allowed for indirect visualization of the anterior chamber and angle. This innovation marked the beginning of modern gonioscopy. The Barkan goniolens became the standard instrument for many decades and was instrumental in the early detection and classification of angle-closure glaucoma.

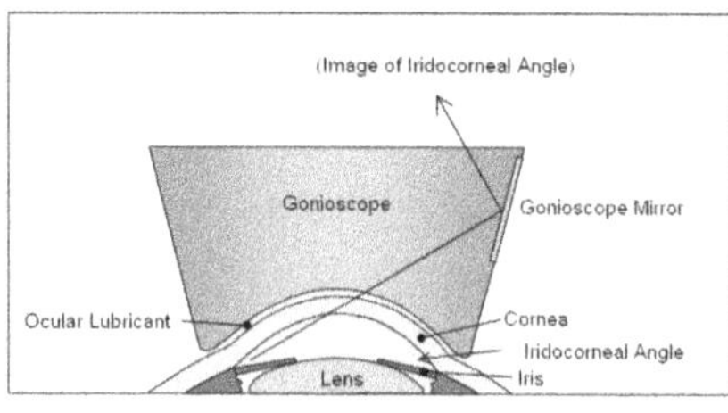

Gonioscopy

Today, gonioscopy is performed using a variety of specialized lenses and instruments, each designed to optimize visualization of the anterior chamber angle under different clinical circumstances. The *Goldmann three-mirror lens* is one of the most widely used instruments in gonioscopy and features three angled mirrors allowing for a comprehensive examination of the anterior chamber angle. It provides high-quality visualization and is particularly useful in cases when a detailed view of the angle is necessary.

Another common instrument is the *Zeiss four-mirror goniolens*, which offers the advantage of providing a panoramic view of the anterior chamber angle without the need to rotate the lens. This feature makes the Zeiss lens more efficient for dynamic gonioscopy to assess the angle under various conditions, such as during compression or manipulation to evaluate the presence of angle-closure mechanisms like synechiae or appositional closure. It is also more portable and easier to use making it a preferred choice in many clinical settings.

The *Posner and Sussman lenses* are also commonly used in gonioscopy. These are handheld four-mirror lenses similar to the Zeiss lens but are smaller in size, allowing for easier manipulation and greater patient comfort. The Sussman lens is favored for its ability to perform gonioscopy in the supine position making it ideal for use in operating rooms or with bedridden individuals.

Ultrasound biomicroscopy (UBM) and *anterior segment optical coherence tomography* (AS-OCT) are advanced imaging modalities that complement traditional gonioscopy by providing high-resolution cross-sectional images of the anterior segment structures. UBM uses high-frequency ultrasound to visualize the anterior chamber angle, ciliary body, and other deep structures which are not easily seen with conventional gonioscopy. AS-OCT, on the other hand, uses light waves to produce detailed images of the anterior chamber angle allowing for precise measurements of angle width and other parameters. These technologies are particularly useful in cases when gonioscopy is inconclusive or when angle structures are difficult to visualize due to corneal opacities or other factors.

Going forward, the development of digital gonioscopy is likely to revolutionize diagnostic capabilities. *Digital gonioscopes* integrating high-resolution cameras with traditional lenses could allow for real-time image capture and documentation, facilitating more accurate diagnosis and the ability to track changes within the anterior chamber over time. These digital systems could also enhance patient education and compliance by viewing images of their own eye structures during evaluations.

Additionally, *robotic and automated gonioscopy systems* are being explored which could standardize the procedure, reduce operator-dependent variability, and increase the accessibility of angle assessments in non-specialized settings. These advancements combined with the integration of artificial intelligence (AI) could lead to more precise, consistent, and automated evaluation of the anterior chamber angle potentially improving early detection and management.

Optical Coherence Tomography

Optical coherence tomography is a non-invasive imaging technology which provides *high-resolution cross-sectional images* of the retina and anterior segment structures of the eye. OCT operates on the principle of low-coherence interferometry, using light waves to capture detailed images of ocular tissues at a micron-scale resolution. This technology has been revolutionary, particularly in the diagnosis and management of retinal disease and glaucoma.

The instrument emits a beam of low-coherence light, typically near-infrared, which penetrates the eye and reflects off various retinal layers. The reflected light is then captured and compared to a reference beam to generate interference patterns. These patterns are processed to create a detailed cross-sectional image of the retina and other ocular structures. OCT can distinguish between different tissue layers allowing for precise measurements of retinal thickness, retinal nerve fiber layer, and the ganglion cell complex (GCC). The technology's resolution is typically in the range of 3 to 15 microns, enabling the detection of minute structural changes which are critical in the early diagnosis of many conditions.

- **Retinal Nerve Fiber Layer & Ganglion Cell Complex**

OCT allows for the quantitative assessment of retinal nerve fiber layer thickness and the ganglion cell complex, which includes the ganglion cell layer and the inner plexiform layer. Thinning of the RNFL and GCC is a hallmark of glaucomatous damage and can be detected by OCT even before visual field defects become apparent. The ability to detect such early changes makes OCT an invaluable tool in the early diagnosis of glaucoma, particularly in patients with ocular hypertension or those at high risk.

In NTG, where IOP is not elevated, OCT can provide critical information by identifying structural damage which may not correlate with IOP levels. The progression of RNFL thinning over time can also be managed utilizing OCT, allowing for the adjustment of treatment plans based on objective measurements of progression.

- **Optic Nerve Head**

OCT provides detailed images of the optic nerve head allowing for the assessment of the neuroretinal rim, optic cup, and important disc parameters. Changes such as increased cup-to-disc ratio, neuroretinal rim thinning, and loss of lamina cribrosa can be visualized and quantified aiding in the diagnosis and management. Its ability to segment the optic nerve into different regions allows for a more nuanced understanding of where glaucomatous optic neuropathy is beginning or occurring, which can help tailor treatment to an individual's specific clinical scenario.

OCT also plays a role in identifying optic disc anomalies that may mimic or exacerbate glaucomatous damage, such as optic disc drusen or tilted discs. In such cases, it can help differentiate between true glaucomatous change and those related to other optic nerve conditions or pathology.

- **Anterior Segment**

OCT is utilized to evaluate structures of the anterior chamber, including the angle. It is particularly useful in angle-closure glaucoma for visualization and assessing the effect of interventions such as laser peripheral iridotomy. It provides a non-contact method with very high resolution and can also be used to accurately corneal thickness, anterior chamber depth, and lens position to the micron. All of which is relevant to each form of glaucoma.

Anterior segment OCT is also valuable in planning and assessing outcomes of surgical interventions, such as trabeculectomy or glaucoma drainage device implantation. It allows for the visualization of bleb formation, aqueous outflow pathways, and the position of implanted devices helping guide postoperative management and identify potential complications early.

Optical Coherence Tomography Angiography

Optical coherence tomography angiography (OCTA) is an advanced imaging modality which provides detailed visualization of the retinal and optic nerve head vasculature *without the need for dye injection*. OCTA builds on the principles of traditional optical coherence tomography by capturing motion contrast from erythrocytes within vessels, allowing for the visualization of microvascular networks.

OCTA has been instrumental in elucidating the relationship between optic nerve head perfusion and glaucomatous damage. Studies have found reduced vessel density in the peripapillary and macular regions correlates with retinal nerve fiber layer thinning and visual field deficits. This suggests microvascular dysfunction likely plays a critical role in glaucoma pathogenesis, particularly in normal-tension glaucoma where IOP is not the primary driving factor.

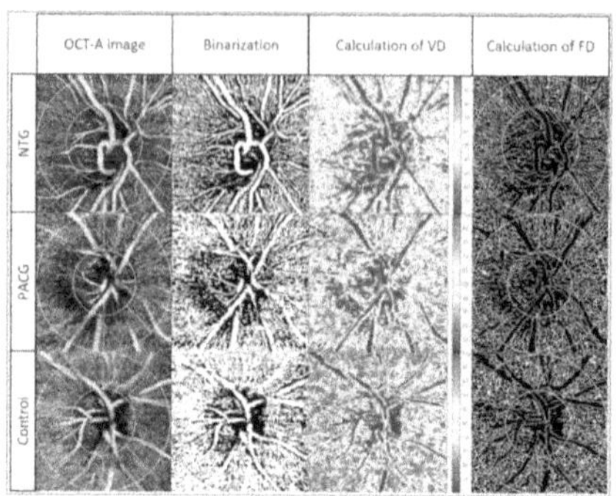

OCTA

It offers several advantages over traditional imaging techniques, including the ability to non-invasively assess microvascular integrity and detect changes in retinal vasculature before structural damage is apparent. Furthermore, OCTA can be used to manage the efficacy of glaucoma treatments by tracking changes in vascular parameters over time. As the technology continues to evolve, it is likely OCTA will become better utilized in diagnosis and management, particularly in early detection of NTG and other forms of glaucoma where vascular factors are implicated.

Swept-Source Optical Coherence Tomography

Swept-source optical coherence tomography (SS-OCT) represents another significant advancement in imaging technology. Unlike traditional spectral-domain OCT (SD-OCT) which uses a broadband light source, SS-OCT employs a *tunable laser which sweeps across a range of wavelengths allowing for deeper tissue penetration and faster acquisition* of images.

SS-OCT provides high-resolution images of the anterior segment, retina, and optic nerve head, with enhanced visualization of deeper structures such as the lamina cribrosa and choroid. This increased depth of imaging is particularly valuable with the lamina cribrosa, a critical site of axonal injury. By enabling detailed assessment of the lamina cribrosa's morphology and biomechanics, SS-OCT offers new insights into structural changes which occur in glaucoma and may help identify individuals at higher risk of progression.

In addition to its application in glaucoma diagnosis, SS-OCT has the potential to improve the assessment of surgical outcomes, such as the patency of filtering blebs following trabeculectomy or the placement of glaucoma drainage devices. As SS-OCT technology becomes more widely available, it is expected to enhance our understanding of glaucoma pathophysiology and refine clinical management.

Visual Fields

Visual field (VF) testing, or perimetry, is an essential diagnostic tool in the evaluation and management of glaucoma providing insight into the functional impact of the condition on vision. Glaucoma being characterized by the progressive loss of retinal ganglion cells and their axons, leads to *characteristic patterns of visual field loss*. Monitoring potential changes over time is vital for assessing disease progression, evaluating the effectiveness of treatment, and adjusting therapeutic strategies.

The history of visual field testing dates to the 19th century when early methods were rudimentary and manually intensive. Hermann Aubert and Richard Förster were among the first to formalize visual field testing in the 1860s, using a hemispherical dome with marked locations to determine a patient's peripheral vision. This method laid the groundwork for modern perimetry. In the mid-20th century, the Goldmann perimeter was introduced which allowed for more precise mapping of the visual field by presenting a moving stimulus on a calibrated screen. The Goldmann perimeter was manual, requiring the examiner to move the stimulus while the patient reported seeing it, making it highly dependent on both the examiner's skill and the patient's responses. Despite these limitations it remained the standard of care for many decades.

Perimetry Techniques

The most widely used device in clinical practice is the *Humphrey Field Analyzer* (HFA), which is considered the gold standard for visual field analysis in glaucoma. The HFA uses a computer-controlled projector to present stimuli at various locations within the visual field, and patients indicate when they see these stimuli by pressing a button. The device measures the differential light sensitivity at multiple points across the field, allowing for the detection of both focal and diffuse characteristic visual field deficits.

HFA provides detailed statistical analyses of the visual field including parameters such as pattern standard deviation (PSD), mean deviation (MD), and the glaucoma hemifield test (GHT), which help differentiate glaucomatous field loss from other types of field loss. Longitudinal monitoring is possible by comparing current visual fields to previous results, enabling the detection of subtle changes over time which may indicate progression.

The *Octopus Perimeter* is another advanced device offering similar capabilities and includes additional features such as cluster analysis and Tendency Oriented Perimetry (TOP), which can reduce testing time enhancing patient comfort and compliance without compromising accuracy.

- **Standard Automated Perimetry** (SAP) is the most commonly used form of perimetry in glaucoma management. SAP involves the use of white light stimuli on a white background, measuring the patient's ability to detect these stimuli across the visual field. It is effective in identifying the characteristic arcuate scotomas and nasal steps associated with glaucoma. However, SAP primarily tests the function of the broader population of retinal ganglion cells and may miss early glaucomatous changes which affect specific subsets of RGCs.

- **Short-Wavelength Automated Perimetry** (SWAP), also known as blue-on-yellow perimetry, enhances the detection of early glaucomatous damage by selectively targeting the blue-sensitive small bistratified ganglion cells in the retina. SWAP uses a blue stimulus on a yellow background, which isolates the response of the short-wavelength cones and their associated ganglion cells. These cells are thought to be more vulnerable in the early stages of glaucoma, making SWAP particularly useful for detecting early functional changes before they become apparent on SAP. However, SWAP is more susceptible to factors such as lens opacities and requires longer testing times which can affect patient compliance.

- **Frequency Doubling Technology** (FDT) Perimetry is another specialized technique used to detect early glaucomatous visual field loss. FDT perimetry presents a low spatial frequency grating that undergoes rapid temporal modulation, creating the illusion of "frequency doubling." This stimulus preferentially activates the magnocellular pathway which is responsible for detecting motion and large objects. The magnocellular cells are believed to be among the first to be affected by glaucomatous damage, making FDT particularly sensitive in detecting early functional loss. FDT is also known for its quick testing time making it ideal for screening purposes, especially in patients who may have difficulty completing longer tests.

- **Microperimetry** represents the next frontier in perimetry, offering a more detailed and localized assessment of retinal sensitivity. Unlike traditional perimetry which maps the visual field relative to a fixation point, microperimetry directly correlates retinal sensitivity with specific locations on the retina using real-time retinal imaging. This is particularly useful in patients with unstable fixation or macular diseases, where traditional perimetry may not provide reliable results. Microperimetry is also valuable for monitoring progression in patients with glaucoma who have coexisting macular pathologies, as it allows for a precise assessment of both conditions simultaneously.

The future of visual field analyses in glaucoma is likely to be shaped by advancements in both hardware and software as well as the integration of artificial intelligence. *Virtual reality (VR)-based perimetry* is an emerging technology which may revolutionize visual field evaluations. VR-based devices can simulate a visual environment in which the patient's visual field can be assessed in a more immersive and patient-friendly manner. These systems have the potential to reduce the physical constraints and discomfort associated with traditional perimetry, particularly for elderly or disabled patients.

AI and machine learning are expected to play a significant role in the evolution of visual field testing. AI algorithms can analyze complex visual field data to identify patterns of glaucomatous damage with greater accuracy, and therefore better predict disease progression. These algorithms can potentially reduce the variability and subjectivity associated with human interpretation of visual field results, leading to more precise and individualized patient management.

Another promising area of development is *multifocal visual evoked potential* (mfVEP), which offers an objective assessment of visual field function by measuring electrical activity in the visual cortex in response to visual stimuli. This method could complement traditional perimetry by providing additional information about the functional integrity of the visual pathway, particularly in cases where standard perimetry is inconclusive or difficult to perform.

Molecular Imaging

Molecular imaging in glaucoma represents a cutting-edge approach to understanding and diagnosing this complex disease at the cellular and molecular levels. Unlike traditional imaging techniques that focus on anatomic structures, molecular imaging allows for the visualization and quantification of specific biological processes within the eye. This technology leverages various modalities, including positron emission tomography (PET), single-photon emission computed tomography (SPECT), and optical coherence tomography combined with *molecular probes*, to target and monitor specific molecules or cellular events involved in glaucoma pathogenesis.

The potential to detect early changes in the retinal ganglion cells, optic nerve head, and surrounding tissues before structural damage becomes apparent can be very powerful. For example, molecular probes that bind to markers of apoptosis or oxidative stress can provide real-time insights into the ongoing degenerative processes in the optic nerve and retina. This enables the early detection of glaucomatous damage even in the absence of significant visual field loss or retinal nerve fiber layer defects.

Additionally, molecular imaging can be used to track the efficacy of neuroprotective therapies by monitoring changes in molecular markers over time. This is particularly important in evaluating the success of experimental treatments aimed at preserving RGCs and their axons. Future advancements in molecular imaging, such as the development of highly specific and sensitive probes, hold promise for personalized glaucoma management allowing for earlier intervention and more targeted therapeutic strategies based on the individual molecular profile of each patient.

Continuous IOP Monitoring

Continuous IOP monitoring represents a significant advancement in glaucoma management, providing *real-time data* on IOP fluctuations which are not captured during standard clinical visits. Traditional methods of IOP measurement, such as tonometry, only offer snapshots of IOP at specific times often missing critical diurnal and nocturnal variations which can strongly contribute to glaucoma progression. Continuous IOP monitoring addresses this limitation by offering dynamic around-the-clock assessment of IOP, leading to a more comprehensive understanding of an individual's IOP profile.

One of the key technologies in this area is the *Sensimed Triggerfish*, a smart contact lens embedded with micro-sensors that measure IOP-related changes in the corneal curvature. This device provides 24-hour IOP monitoring, capturing data that can reveal nocturnal spikes or other fluctuations which might not be detected during office hours. The data is wirelessly transmitted to a recorder allowing for detailed analysis.

Another emerging technology involves implantable IOP sensors like the *Implandata EyeMate* system, which is implanted during cataract or glaucoma surgery. This device provides direct IOP measurements enabling real-time monitoring with remote data transmission. These sensors offer high precision and eliminate the variability associated with external measurements.

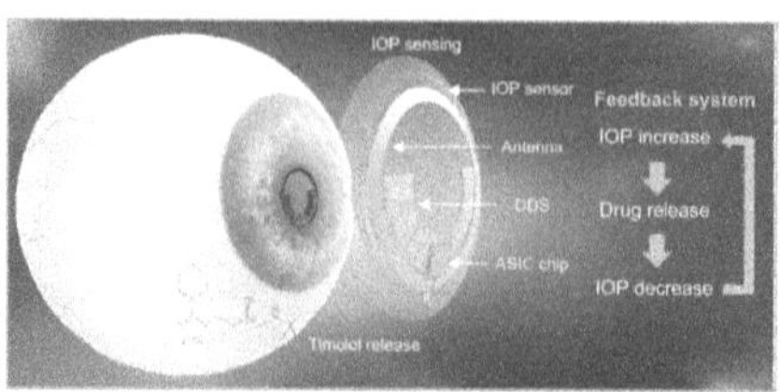

IOP Sensing Contact Lens

The future of continuous IOP monitoring may include even more sophisticated wearable devices, further miniaturization of sensors, and integration with artificial intelligence algorithms to predict glaucoma progression and optimize personalized treatment plans. The technology is poised to revolutionize glaucoma care by enabling early intervention and more effective management based on comprehensive real-time IOP data.

Biomarkers

The search for reliable biomarkers in glaucoma has been an area of intense research, driven by the need for objective measures which can aid in early diagnosis, monitor progression, and predict therapeutic response. Biomarkers can be broadly categorized into *structural, functional, and molecular markers*, each offering unique insights into the disease process.

- **Structural**

Structural biomarkers include parameters such as retinal nerve fiber layer thickness, ganglion cell complex thickness, and optic nerve head morphology, all of which are routinely assessed using OCT. Reductions in these structural metrics are indicative of glaucomatous damage and have been shown to correlate with visual field loss.

Recent advancements in imaging technology have enabled the identification of more subtle structural biomarkers, such as changes in the lamina cribrosa or choroidal thickness, which may precede overt damage to the RNFL or GCC. These early structural changes hold promise as biomarkers for identifying individuals at risk of glaucoma progression even sooner.

- **Functional**

Functional biomarkers primarily involve visual field testing, with standard automated perimetry being the most utilized method. However, functional changes often lag behind structural damage, leading to the development of more sensitive methods such as frequency-doubling technology perimetry and short-wavelength automated perimetry.

Emerging functional biomarkers include assessments of retinal ganglion cell function, such as pattern electroretinography (pERG) and photopic negative response (PhNR), which may detect early glaucomatous changes at the level of the retinal ganglion cells before additional pathology become apparent. These advanced functional modalities provide a more nuanced understanding of how glaucoma affects retinal function and may offer a means of detection at a much earlier stage.

- **Molecular**

Molecular biomarkers involve the detection of specific proteins, metabolites, or genetic markers in ocular tissues or fluids. For example, elevated levels of matrix metalloproteinases (MMPs) and pro-inflammatory cytokines in the aqueous humor have been associated with glaucoma progression, particularly in cases of secondary glaucoma such as uveitic glaucoma.

Genetic markers, including single nucleotide polymorphisms in genes such as MYOC, OPTN, and CYP1B1, have been identified as risk factors for glaucoma and may serve as biomarkers for predicting disease susceptibility or response to treatment. Advances in proteomics and metabolomics are likely to uncover additional molecular biomarkers which can be used to stratify individuals based on their risk of progression and guide personalized treatment strategies.

Artificial Intelligence

The future role of artificial intelligence in glaucoma management is set to be transformative by enabling more precise, personalized, and proactive care. AI, particularly through machine learning and deep learning algorithms, has the *ability to process and analyze vast amounts of clinical data such as optical coherence tomography, visual fields, and patient history far more efficiently* than what is possible today. This capability allows AI to detect subtle patterns and early signs of glaucoma which may elude even the most experienced clinicians, facilitating earlier diagnosis and intervention.

AI algorithms will integrate data from multiple imaging modalities to provide a more comprehensive risk assessment.

By evaluating parameters like retinal nerve fiber layer thickness, optic nerve head morphology, visual field patterns, and other pertinent factors, AI can enhance the sensitivity and specificity of glaucoma detection. This integrated approach not only improves diagnostic accuracy but also helps in stratifying patients according to their risk of progression.

Furthermore, it has the potential to revolutionize glaucoma monitoring over time. AI-driven tools can continuously analyze longitudinal data to better predict progression and identify individuals at higher risk of rapid deterioration. This predictive capability allows for timely adjustments in treatment, potentially preventing vision loss.

Looking ahead, the integration of AI with telemedicine and wearable technology for continuous intraocular pressure monitoring could further enhance patient care, enabling remote management and more frequent monitoring.

Chapter 7
Medical Management

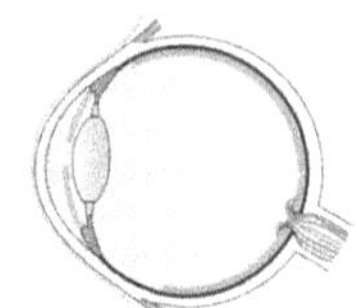

Glaucoma management encompasses a broad spectrum of therapeutic strategies aimed at lowering intraocular pressure, the primary modifiable risk factor in glaucoma. The goal is to prevent or slow down the progression of optic neuropathy and preserve visual function. Treatment modalities include pharmacologic therapies, laser procedures, and surgical interventions, each with specific indications, mechanisms of action, and potential complications.

Pharmacologic Treatment

Pharmacologic therapy is often first-line treatment, particularly in cases of primary open-angle glaucoma and ocular hypertension. The primary goal of pharmacologic treatment is to lower intraocular pressure by either reducing the production of aqueous humor or increasing its outflow. There are several classes of medications used in glaucoma management, each with distinct mechanisms of action, efficacy profiles, and potential adverse effects.

Prostaglandin Analogues

Prostaglandin analogues are the most prescribed class of glaucoma medications due to their efficacy, once-daily dosing, and relatively favorable side effect profile. They are a cornerstone in the management of primary open-angle glaucoma as well as ocular hypertension, and include *latanoprost*, *bimatoprost*, *travoprost*, and *tafluprost*. Prostaglandin analogues typically lower IOP by 25-35% from baseline, making them highly effective as monotherapy or in combination with other IOP-lowering agents. More recently, latanoprostene bunod, a dual-action drug is available which combines latanoprost with a nitric oxide donor. Latanoprostene bunod has a mechanism of action like traditional prostaglandin analogues, however, it also enhances trabecular outflow by relaxing the trabecular meshwork through the release of nitric oxide. Recent research has shown it may also increase ocular perfusion, which can be beneficial in normal tension glaucoma in individuals with underlying circulatory insufficiency.

The primary mechanism of action of prostaglandin analogues involves *enhancing the outflow of aqueous humor through the uveoscleral pathway*, a secondary drainage route within the eye. They are lipid compounds that naturally occur in the body and play a role in various physiological processes, including inflammation, vasodilation, and regulation of smooth muscle tone. In the context of glaucoma treatment, synthetic analogues of prostaglandins are designed to mimic the activity of the naturally occurring prostaglandin F2α.

Upon topical application, prostaglandin analogues bind to prostaglandin F (FP) receptors located in the ciliary muscle and other ocular tissues. Activation of these receptors initiates a cascade of intracellular signaling events that lead to the remodeling of the extracellular matrix within the ciliary muscle and adjacent sclera. This remodeling process involves the upregulation of matrix metalloproteinases, enzymes that degrade extracellular matrix components such as collagen and proteoglycans. As a result, the uveoscleral outflow pathway becomes less resistant allowing for increased aqueous humor drainage from the eye.

The enhanced uveoscleral outflow effectively reduces intraocular pressure which is the goal in slowing the progression of glaucomatous optic neuropathy. Prostaglandin analogues are particularly effective in lowering pressure due to their potent action and prolonged duration of effect, allowing for once-daily dosing. Additionally, they have a favorable side effect profile, with the most common adverse effects being localized to the ocular surface such as conjunctival hyperemia, increased eyelash growth, and changes in iris pigmentation.

The remodeling of the extracellular matrix in the ciliary muscle and sclera is a dynamic and reversible process, which contributes to the sustained reduction in IOP observed with continued use of prostaglandin analogues. Furthermore, these agents have been shown to be effective in a broad range of individuals including those who may not respond adequately to other classes of IOP-lowering medications.

Beta-Adrenergic Antagonists

Beta-blockers are a well-established class of medications used in the management of glaucoma, particularly for lowering intraocular pressure in conditions such as primary open-angle glaucoma and ocular hypertension. The primary mechanism of action of beta-blockers involves the *reduction of aqueous humor production by the ciliary body*, thereby decreasing intraocular pressure to prevent further optic neuropathy and progression.

Beta-blockers exert their effects by blocking beta-adrenergic receptors, specifically beta-2 adrenergic receptors, which are predominant on the ciliary body epithelium. Under normal physiological conditions, activation of these receptors by catecholamines such as norepinephrine stimulates adenylate cyclase activity, leading to an increase in cyclic adenosine monophosphate (cAMP) levels within the ciliary epithelium. Elevated cAMP levels promote aqueous humor production through the activation of protein kinase A (PKA), which enhances the secretion of aqueous humor from the ciliary processes.

When beta-blockers are applied topically to the eye, they inhibit the beta-adrenergic receptors on the ciliary epithelium leading to a decrease in cAMP production. This reduction in cAMP activity results in a downregulation of aqueous humor formation, effectively lowering IOP. The decrease in aqueous humor production reduces the amount of fluid within the anterior chamber of the eye, thereby lowering intraocular pressure.

Several beta-blockers are commonly used in the treatment of glaucoma, with *timolol* being one of the most widely prescribed due to its efficacy and favorable safety profile, and often lowering pressure by approximately 20-25%. Other beta-blockers include *betaxolol, levobunolol,* and *metipranolol,* each with varying degrees of receptor selectivity and side effect profiles. Betaxolol, for instance, is a selective beta-1 adr

energic receptor blocker and is often preferred in patients with pulmonary conditions as it is less likely to induce bronchoconstriction, a common side effect associated with non-selective beta-blockers like timolol.

The efficacy of beta-blockers in lowering IOP typically lasts for 12 to 24 hours, allowing for twice-daily dosing for most individuals. However, the effectiveness of beta-blockers may diminish over time due to tachyphylaxis, where the receptors become less responsive to the drug. Additionally, systemic absorption of beta-blockers through the nasolacrimal duct can lead to *systemic adverse effects, such as bradycardia, hypotension, and bronchospasm,* particularly in susceptible individuals.

Despite these potential drawbacks, beta-blockers remain a viable option in the pharmacological management of glaucoma, often used as first-line therapy or in combination with other intraocular pressure lowering agents such as prostaglandin analogues. Their well-documented efficacy in reducing aqueous humor production and lowering IOP, along with their relatively low cost, make them very popular in glaucoma management.

Alpha-2 Adrenergic Agonists

Alpha-2 adrenergic agonists are an important class of medications used in the treatment of glaucoma, particularly in primary open-angle glaucoma and ocular hypertension. The mechanism of action of alpha-2 agonists primarily involves dual actions, by *reducing aqueous humor production and enhancing uveoscleral outflow.*

They achieve their therapeutic effect by selectively stimulating alpha-2 receptors located on the ciliary body epithelium. These receptors, when activated, inhibit adenylate cyclase activity leading to a decrease in cyclic adenosine monophosphate levels within the ciliary epithelium. Since cAMP is a key mediator in the production of aqueous humor, its reduction leads to a decrease in aqueous thereby lowering pressure.

Additionally, alpha-2 agonists have been shown to increase uveoscleral outflow, the secondary drainage pathway for aqueous humor. This effect is believed to result from the contraction of the ciliary muscle and changes in the extracellular matrix which create a less resistant pathway for the aqueous humor to exit the eye. By simultaneously reducing inflow and enhancing outflow of aqueous humor, alpha-2 agonists provide a comprehensive approach to management.

Brimonidine is the most used alpha-2 agonist in glaucoma management due to its high selectivity for its receptors and favorable safety profile. It is often preferred because it has a lower risk of systemic side effects, compared to earlier less selective alpha-adrenergic agonists like apraclonidine. However, it is important to note some individuals may experience adverse effects such as allergic conjunctivitis, dry mouth, and fatigue. The effectiveness of brimonidine in lowering pressure typically lasts for about 8 to 12 hours, necessitating multiple doses per day, usually two to three times daily.

Another notable aspect of alpha-2 adrenergic agonists is their *potential neuroprotective effects*, which are of particular interest in glaucoma management. Experimental studies have suggested brimonidine may help protect retinal ganglion cells from apoptosis through mechanisms which involve modulation of glutamate toxicity, reduction of oxidative stress, and inhibition of neuroinflammation. While these neuroprotective effects are still under investigation and not yet fully understood, they represent a promising avenue for additional therapeutic benefits of alpha-adrenergic agonists beyond pressure reduction alone.

In terms of systemic safety, alpha-2 adrenergic agonists are generally well tolerated, but they can cross the blood-brain barrier potentially leading to *central nervous system effects such as drowsiness and hypotension* especially in elderly patients. Although extremely rare, *depression and suicidal ideations* have also been known to occur due to *alpha-2 agonists link to central nervous system depression*. Therefore, careful monitoring and patient selection is important when prescribing these medications, particularly in those with cardiovascular conditions. In fact, brimonidine is contraindicated in children under 2 years-old also due to the risk of central nervous system depression.

Carbonic Anhydrase Inhibitors

Carbonic anhydrase inhibitors (CAIs) are an important class of sulfa-based medications in the treatment of glaucoma, particularly for lowering intraocular pressure in primary open-angle glaucoma and ocular hypertension. These drugs *target the enzyme carbonic anhydrase* which is highly expressed within the ciliary body of the eye, specifically in the non-pigmented ciliary epithelium. The primary mechanism of action of CAIs involves the inhibition of this enzyme, thereby *reducing the production of aqueous humor* leading to a decrease in pressure.

Carbonic anhydrase plays an essential role in the production of aqueous humor. This enzyme catalyzes the reversible reaction that converts carbon dioxide and water into bicarbonate ions and protons.

$$CO_2 + H_2O => HCO_3^- + H^+$$

In the ciliary body bicarbonate ions are key for the transport of sodium and water into the posterior chamber, contributing to the osmotic gradient that drives the secretion of aqueous humor. By facilitating this ionic exchange, carbonic anhydrase supports the continuous production of aqueous humor.

CAIs such as *acetazolamide* (oral), *dorzolamide* or *brinzolamide* (topical), inhibit the activity of carbonic anhydrase which is abundant in the ciliary epithelium. Inhibition of this enzyme reduces the production of bicarbonate ions leading to a decrease in the transport of sodium and water into the posterior chamber. As a result, the production of aqueous humor is diminished reducing intraocular pressure.

Dorzolamide and brinzolamide are widely used for management of glaucoma due to their targeted action within the eye and low incidence of systemic side effects. They are often used as part of combination therapy, especially in patients who require additional pressure reduction beyond what is achieved with first-line therapies like prostaglandin analogues or beta-blockers. Topical CAIs are generally well-tolerated, but some individuals may experience ocular side effects such as stinging, burning, and a bitter taste. These effects are usually mild and transient.

Systemic CAIs like acetazolamide are generally reserved for *short-term or acute management scenarios*, such as in the treatment of acute angle-closure glaucoma or when rapid pressure reduction is necessary. They inhibit carbonic anhydrase throughout the body leading to a more pronounced reduction in aqueous humor production. However, their use is limited by potential *adverse effects including metabolic acidosis, electrolyte imbalance, paresthesia, and gastrointestinal disturbances*. This necessitates careful patient selection and monitoring, particularly in individuals with pre-existing renal, hepatic, or respiratory conditions.

Rho Kinase Inhibitors

Rho kinase inhibitors represent a relatively new and innovative class of medications offering a unique mechanism of action distinct from traditional intraocular pressure lowering therapies. These agents specifically *target the Rho/Rho-associated protein kinase (ROCK) signaling pathway* which plays a critical role in regulating various cellular processes, including cytoskeletal dynamics, cell contractility, and extracellular matrix remodeling. By inhibiting this pathway, they exert multiple effects which collectively lower pressure and also possibly provide neuroprotective benefits, making them an exciting addition to the therapeutic arsenal.

The Rho/Rho kinase pathway is involved in the *regulation of contractile tone and stiffness of the trabecular meshwork* and surrounding juxtacanalicular tissue. Activation of this pathway leads to increased actin-myosin contraction and elevated extracellular matrix deposition, both of which contribute to increased outflow resistance and higher IOP. Rho kinase inhibitors work by inhibiting Rho kinase, leading to relaxation of the trabecular meshwork cells and a decrease in the stiffness of the extracellular matrix. This relaxation facilitates the outflow of aqueous humor through the trabecular meshwork thereby lowering pressure.

In addition to enhancing trabecular outflow, Rho kinase inhibitors have been shown to *reduce episcleral venous pressure*, which further contributes to IOP reduction. Some studies have also suggested they may decrease aqueous humor production, although this effect is less pronounced compared to their primary action on the trabecular meshwork.

ROCK inhibitors are used as part of the pharmacological management of glaucoma, particularly in cases where traditional therapies may not provide adequate pressure control. *Netarsudil* is the first Rho kinase inhibitor approved and can be used as monotherapy, or in combination with other pressure-lowering agents such as prostaglandin analogues or beta-blockers.

The most common adverse effects of Rho kinase inhibitors are related to their vasodilatory effects on the ocular surface, which can lead to *conjunctival injection* or hyperemia. This is thought to result from the relaxation of smooth muscle within the walls of conjunctival vessels, a mechanism similar to the effect on the trabecular meshwork. Other ocular effects may include mild *corneal verticillata and subconjunctival hemorrhages*, both of which are generally asymptomatic and reversible upon discontinuation of treatment.

Cholinergic Agonists

Cholinergic agonists, miotics such as *pilocarpine*, are a long-standing class of medications. Pilocarpine works by directly stimulating parasympathetic muscarinic receptors, primarily the M3 subtype, in the ciliary muscle and iris sphincter muscle. This activation induces *contraction of the ciliary muscle which increases aqueous outflow* through the trabecular meshwork. Additionally, pilocarpine creates *miosis which helps open the anterior chamber angle*, reducing risk of angle closure in individuals with narrow angles.

Clinically, pilocarpine is most often used in acute angle-closure glaucoma, where its rapid action is beneficial in quickly lowering pressure and potentially relieving angle closure before surgical or laser intervention. It may also be used in primary open-angle glaucoma, though its use has decreased in favor of newer more efficacious agents with fewer adverse effects.

Common side effects include blurred vision, particularly in low-light conditions, headache or brow ache due to ciliary muscle contraction, and transient myopia. There is also an increased risk of retinal detachment. It is contraindicated in patients with uveitis, as it can exacerbate inflammation. Despite its profile, it remains an important therapeutic option in certain clinical scenarios.

Adenosine Receptor Agonists

Adenosine receptor agonists represent an emerging class of therapeutic agents, leveraging the modulatory effects of adenosine on intraocular pressure and neuroprotection. Adenosine is a *naturally occurring nucleoside* which plays a critical role in various physiological processes, including regulation of ocular blood flow and aqueous dynamics. The eye expresses several adenosine receptor subtypes, among which A1 and A3 receptors have received particular interest for their potential in glaucoma management.

Their primary mechanism of action involves activation of A1 receptors located in the trabecular meshwork and ciliary body. When activated, these receptors *enhance outflow of aqueous* through the trabecular meshwork by promoting cytoskeletal changes and modulating the extracellular matrix, leading to increased outflow facility and reduced pressure. Additionally, A1 receptor activation in the ciliary body has been shown to *decrease aqueous humor production* further contributing to pressure reduction.

Beyond their effects on IOP, adenosine receptor agonists also exhibit *neuroprotective properties* through the activation of A3 receptors. Activation of A3 receptors on retinal ganglion cells and glial cells trigger intracellular signaling pathways which reduce oxidative stress, inhibit apoptosis, and promote cell survival. These neuroprotective effects are particularly important as RGC degeneration is the hallmark of glaucomatous progression.

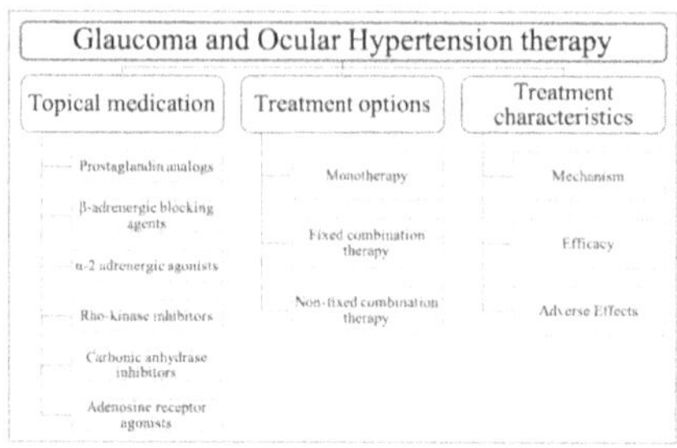

Pharmacologic Options

Non-IOP Lowering Therapies

There have been significant strides made in understanding the complex pathophysiology of glaucomatous optic neuropathy. While elevated intraocular pressure remains a major risk factor, the mechanical theory fails to explain cases of ocular hypertension without neuropathy and does not provide rationale for normal-tension glaucoma. In fact, the *Ocular Hypertension Treatment Study reported over 90% of individuals with elevated pressure did not progress to glaucoma when followed over a 5-year period*. This suggests factors beyond intraocular pressure contribute to glaucomatous damage.

- **Neuroprotection**

Neuroprotection in glaucoma is a rapidly evolving area of research aimed at directly preserving retinal ganglion cells and their axons, which are progressively damaged in glaucomatous optic neuropathy. Several neuroprotective agents are currently undergoing clinical trials to assess their potential in preventing or slowing glaucomatous neuropathy.

NT-501, an implantable device which delivers ciliary neurotrophic factor (CNTF), has shown promise in preserving visual acuity and visual fields. CNTF is a neurotrophic factor which supports the survival of neurons, including RGCs, and the NT-501 device ensures sustained delivery of CNTF directly to the retina potentially offering long-term neuroprotection.

Recombinant human nerve growth factor (rhNGF) is another neuroprotective agent under investigation. RhNGF has also been shown to promote the survival and regeneration of RGCs. In phase 1b trials, rhNGF has demonstrated safety and potential efficacy in primary open-angle glaucoma making it a promising candidate for further development.

Citicoline, a naturally occurring phospholipid precursor, has gained attention as well. Citicoline enhances the synthesis of phosphatidylcholine, a key component of cell membranes, supporting neuronal integrity. Oral citicoline supplementation has been shown to improve retinal function and neural conduction along the visual pathway as evidenced by improvements in pattern electroretinogram and visual evoked potential (VEP) measurements. The ongoing Phase IV clinical trial (NCT03046693) aims to further evaluate the efficacy of citicoline.

Other notable neuroprotective strategies include *memantine*, an NMDA receptor antagonist, which may prevent glutamate-induced excitotoxicity. *Brimonidine*, an alpha-2 adrenergic agonist with demonstrated neuroprotective properties through the reduction of glutamate release and enhancement of neurotrophic factor expression, has been a drug of focus for several years. Rho kinase inhibitors, like *netarsudil*, are being further explored for their dual mechanism of action which includes both IOP reduction and potential neuroprotection by modulating the cytoskeleton and reducing stress on the optic nerve head.

Despite these advances, translating neuroprotective therapies from the laboratory to clinical practice remains a significant challenge. Ongoing research and clinical trials continue to explore these promising therapies, with the goal of integrating neuroprotection as standard of care.

- **Ocular Perfusion**

The vascular theory supports glaucomatous neuropathy being driven by *reduced ocular perfusion pressure, impaired vascular autoregulation, and/or disrupted neurovascular coupling*. These abnormalities can lead to insufficient blood flow to the optic nerve head, resulting in ischemic oxidative stress and triggering the apoptosis of retinal ganglion cells. Reduced ocular perfusion pressure has been identified as a significant risk factor for the prevalence, incidence, and progression of glaucoma, emphasizing the role of vascular health in its pathogenesis.

Vascular endothelial dysfunction is increasingly recognized as a contributing factor in glaucoma. The vascular endothelium plays a key role in regulating microcirculation through the release of vasoactive factors, such as nitric oxide, endothelin-1, and vascular endothelial growth factor. Dysregulation of these factors has been implicated in the pathophysiology.

Nitric oxide is a potent vasodilator which helps maintain normal blood flow within the ocular microcirculation. In glaucoma patients, reduced levels of NO have been associated with decreased vasodilatation and increased vasoconstriction, leading to compromised blood flow to the optic nerve head. Therapeutic strategies aimed at enhancing NO bioavailability are being explored to improve ocular blood flow and protect against glaucomatous damage. For example, L-arginine supplementation, a precursor to NO synthesis is under investigation for its potential to increase NO levels and improve ocular perfusion.

Endothelin-1 is a potent vasoconstrictor that has been found at elevated levels in both the plasma and aqueous humor. ET-1 can induce significant constriction of the vasculature supplying the optic nerve, reducing blood flow and contributing to ischemia and progressive optic neuropathy. Researchers are studying endothelin receptor antagonists, such as *bosentan*, for their ability to block the effects of ET-1 potentially reducing vasoconstriction and improving ocular blood flow.

Vascular endothelial growth factor is another critical factor in glaucoma pathogenesis, particularly in the context of hypoxia. VEGF is upregulated in hypoxic environments and has also been found at elevated levels in the aqueous humor. While VEGF promotes angiogenesis and is essential for maintaining vascular health, its *overexpression can lead to pathological neovascularization* contributing to secondary glaucoma, specifically neovascular glaucoma. Anti-VEGF therapies, like *ranibizumab* and *bevacizumab*, are being explored for their potential to control neovascularization and reduce risk.

- **Mitochondrial Protection**

Mitochondrial dysfunction has emerged as a critical factor in the pathogenesis of glaucoma, contributing to the degeneration of retinal ganglion cells. Mitochondria play the key role in intracellular energy production through oxidative phosphorylation. However, this process also generates reactive oxygen species as byproducts, which under normal circumstances are kept in check by the cell's antioxidant defenses. In glaucoma, the delicate balance between *ROS production and antioxidant defense can be disrupted* leading to oxidative stress, a state where excessive ROS creates significant cellular and mitochondrial damage ultimately resulting in retinal ganglion cell apoptosis.

The vulnerability of RGCs to mitochondrial dysfunction and oxidative stress is heightened by their high metabolic demand and complex structure, which relies on efficient energy production and intracellular transport. As glaucoma progresses, the accumulation of mitochondrial damage can impair and reduce ATP production triggering the release of pro-apoptotic factors, all of which contribute to RGC death and optic neuropathy.

Mitochondria-targeted antioxidants have emerged as a promising therapeutic strategy aimed at mitigating oxidative stress and preserving mitochondrial function. Unlike traditional antioxidants that act more broadly within a cell, these agents are specifically designed to accumulate within the mitochondria, where they can directly neutralize ROS and protect against progressive damage.

MitoQ is one such mitochondria-targeted antioxidant which has shown significant promise in preclinical studies. It is composed of a *ubiquinone/coenzyme Q10 moiety* linked to a triphenylphosphonium cation, which enables it to selectively accumulate in the mitochondria. Once inside the mitochondria, MitoQ acts as a potent ROS scavenger neutralizing free radicals and preventing oxidative damage that can lead to mitochondrial dysfunction and RGC death. Preclinical models have demonstrated it can protect against RGC loss, preserve optic nerve integrity, and maintain visual function suggesting its potential as a viable neuroprotective therapy.

Another promising mitochondria-targeted antioxidant is *SkQ1* (plastoquinonyl-decyl-triphenylphosphonium), which also accumulates within the mitochondria due to its lipophilic cationic structure. It is derived from plastoquinone, a naturally occurring antioxidant found in plants, and is designed to protect mitochondrial membranes from oxidative damage. In animal models of glaucoma, SkQ1 has been shown to reduce ROS levels, prevent RGC apoptosis, and also preserve visual function. The neuroprotective effects are believed to arise from its ability to stabilize mitochondrial membranes, reduce mitochondrial swelling, and prevent the release of cytochrome c, a key factor in the intrinsic apoptotic pathway.

Beyond mitochondria-targeted antioxidants, other strategies aimed at preserving mitochondrial function are also under investigation. These include agents that enhance mitochondrial biogenesis, such as peroxisome proliferator-activated receptor gamma coactivator 1-alpha, *PGC-1α activators, which promote the formation of new mitochondria* and improve cellular resilience to oxidative stress.

Additionally, mitochondrial uncouplers that mildly dissipate the proton gradient across the mitochondrial membrane are being explored for their ability to reduce ROS production without impairing ATP synthesis. *Pharmacological chaperones* that stabilize mitochondrial proteins, and *gene therapies* designed to enhance the expression of mitochondrial antioxidants or repair defective mitochondrial DNA, are also being investigated as potential neuroprotective strategies.

- **Antioxidants**

Antioxidant therapy represents a vital approach targeting oxidative stress which contributes to retinal ganglion cell degeneration and glaucomatous optic neuropathy. Oxidative stress arises from an imbalance between the production of reactive oxygen species and the eye's antioxidant defenses, leading to cellular damage, inflammation, and apoptosis. Excessive ROS generated in the retina and optic nerve head can exacerbate neurodegenerative processes and contribute to the progressive nature of uncontrolled glaucoma.

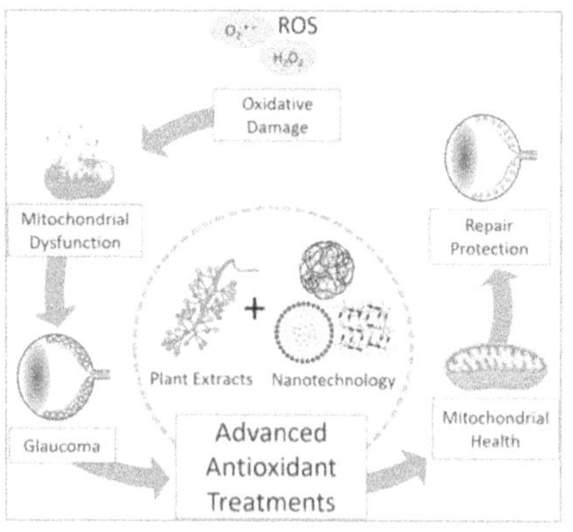

Oxidative Stress & Glaucoma

Several antioxidants have been well known for their neuroprotective potential, including *vitamin C* (ascorbic acid), *vitamin E* (alpha-tocopherol), and *glutathione*. They function by neutralizing free radicals, thereby preventing lipid peroxidation and protecting cellular membranes from oxidative damage. Vitamin C, a water-soluble antioxidant, is particularly effective in scavenging ROS in the aqueous humor where it can directly protect the trabecular meshwork. Vitamin E, a fat-soluble antioxidant, protects lipid-rich cellular structures such as the myelin sheath surrounding optic nerve fibers. Glutathione, a tripeptide composed of glutamine, cysteine, and glycine, is an important intracellular antioxidant which helps maintain the redox balance within RGCs and supports the detoxification of ROS.

Among promising antioxidants, *coenzyme Q10* (CoQ10) has gained significant attention due to its dual role as an electron transporter in the mitochondrial respiratory chain and as an antioxidant. CoQ10 is a lipophilic molecule naturally found in the inner mitochondrial membrane, where it facilitates the transfer of electrons between complex I and complex III during oxidative phosphorylation, a process essential for ATP energy production. In addition to its role in energy metabolism, CoQ10 also acts as a potent antioxidant scavenging ROS and preventing oxidative damage within the mitochondria.

Supplementation with CoQ10 has shown promising results in the context of glaucoma. Studies have demonstrated it can improve visual function and reduce oxidative stress in individuals with primary open-angle glaucoma. Moreover, its neuroprotective effects may be potentiated when used in combination with other antioxidants or IOP-lowering therapies. For instance, formulations combining CoQ10 with vitamin E or other antioxidants may provide a synergistic effect, offering more comprehensive protection against oxidative damage. Additionally, ongoing research is exploring the potential of analogs and derivatives, which may offer improved bioavailability and efficacy in targeting mitochondrial dysfunction.

Chapter 8

Laser Therapy

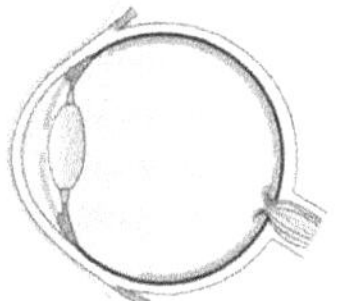

Laser Therapy

Various laser treatments play a significant role, particularly in cases where pharmacologic treatment alone is insufficient to achieve target IOP. Laser procedures offer the advantage of being less invasive than surgery, with relatively quick recovery times and potential for repeat treatments. Two of the most utilized laser treatments in glaucoma management are *Selective Laser Trabeculoplasty* (SLT) and *Laser Peripheral Iridotomy* (LPI).

Selective Laser Trabeculoplasty

Selective Laser Trabeculoplasty is a highly effective procedure employed to lower intraocular pressure in patients with open-angle glaucoma, particularly primary open-angle glaucoma, ocular hypertension, and pseudoexfoliative glaucoma. It specifically targets the trabecular meshwork, the principal site for aqueous outflow, to enhance drainage and reduce IOP.

Unlike earlier forms of laser trabeculoplasty, such as Argon Laser Trabeculoplasty (ALT), SLT is distinct in its "selective" nature and *precisely targets pigmented trabecular cells* while sparing adjacent non-pigmented cells from significant thermal damage. This selectivity is important in minimizing tissue injury and preserving integrity of the trabecular meshwork, allowing for the procedure to be safely repeated if necessary.

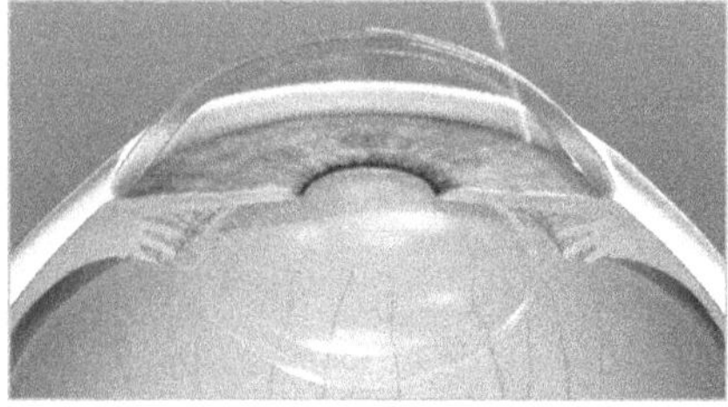

SLT Targeting Trabeculum

SLT employs a 532-nm frequency-doubled Nd:YAG laser to deliver short, low-energy pulses to the trabecular meshwork. The laser energy is absorbed by melanin within the pigmented trabecular cells, leading to a process known as selective photothermolysis. This targeted thermal effect triggers a biological response without causing widespread coagulative damage, as seen in ALT. The photothermolytic effect initiates a cascade of events, including remodeling of the extracellular matrix and increased activity of macrophages within the trabecular meshwork. These changes enhance outflow of aqueous humor by reducing resistance within the trabecular meshwork, leading to a subsequent decrease in IOP. The cellular and molecular mechanisms involved in SLT also include upregulation of cytokines and matrix metalloproteinases which contribute to the degradation of extracellular matrix components and further facilitate aqueous outflow.

It is indicated for individuals with primary open-angle glaucoma, ocular hypertension, and pseudoexfoliative glaucoma, particularly those who require additional IOP reduction beyond what is achieved with pharmacologic therapy or for those who are intolerant or non-adherent to medications. It can also be utilized as an initial primary treatment, or as a repeat procedure in cases where the initial IOP reduction diminishes over time. Clinical studies have shown SLT can lower IOP by 20-30% from baseline, with its efficacy comparable to that of prostaglandin analogues, which are among the most potent IOP-lowering medications available.

The ability of SLT to achieve significant IOP reduction without causing substantial damage to the trabecular meshwork makes it an attractive option for long-term glaucoma management. It is minimally invasive, generally well-tolerated and associated with minimal discomfort. Additionally, because it does not cause extensive scarring of the trabecular meshwork, it can be repeated safely providing sustained IOP control over time.

While it is generally considered safe, it is not entirely free from potential complications. Some individuals may experience transient ocular discomfort, conjunctival hyperemia, or a mild anterior uveitis (iritis) following the procedure. These effects are typically mild and self-limiting, resolving within a few days to weeks with minimal intervention. However, in rare cases, SLT can lead to a pressure spike which usually occurs within the first few hours post-procedure. This pressure spike can be managed with topical medications and typically resolves without long-term consequences.

Given the potential for inflammation and IOP spikes, patients undergoing SLT should be reassessed in the immediate post-procedure period. The use of anti-inflammatory medications such as topical corticosteroids or non-steroidal anti-inflammatory drugs (NSAIDs) is often recommended to reduce inflammation and prevent possible discomfort. Overall, the risk of significant complications with SLT is low making it a safe and effective option.

Laser Peripheral Iridotomy

Laser Peripheral Iridotomy is a well-established procedure used to treat narrow-angle glaucoma and prevent angle-closure glaucoma. LPI *creates a small full-thickness opening in the peripheral iris*, providing an alternative pathway for aqueous humor to flow directly from the posterior chamber to the anterior chamber. This bypasses the pupillary block, a condition where the iris is pushed forward against the trabecular meshwork obstructing aqueous outflow and leading to a rise in intraocular pressure.

The procedure is typically performed using an Nd:YAG laser, or less commonly an argon laser. The laser energy is precisely focused to create a full-thickness iridotomy usually located in the superior or temporal peripheral iris. It is minimally invasive, quick, and generally performed in an outpatient or office setting under topical anesthesia minimizing discomfort.

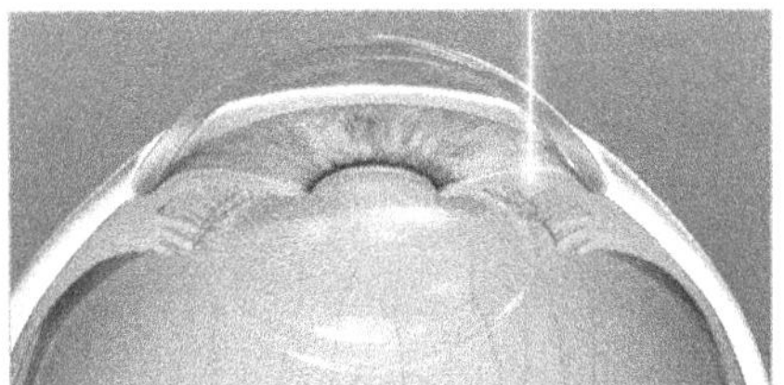

LPI Targeting Peripheral Iris

LPI is indicated for individuals with acute angle-closure glaucoma, chronic angle-closure glaucoma, and those with anatomically narrow angles who are at risk of developing angle closure. It is also frequently performed prophylactically in patients with narrow angles to prevent the development of angle-closure glaucoma, or in the fellow eye of individuals who have already experienced an acute angle-closure event.

In cases of acute angle-closure, a medical emergency, immediate LPI is highly effective in rapidly lowering IOP and alleviating symptoms such as severe ocular pain, headache, nausea, and visual disturbances. By relieving the pupillary block, it can prevent irreversible optic neuropathy and potential atrophy which could otherwise result from sustained elevated IOP. In chronic angle-closure glaucoma, LPI can reduce and stabilize IOP preventing further angle closure and slow progression.

While LPI is generally considered safe and effective, it is also not without potential complications. Some individuals may experience transient ocular discomfort, mild anterior chamber inflammation, or a transient increase in IOP following the procedure. These issues are typically mild and can be managed with anti-inflammatory medications such as topical corticosteroids, and IOP-lowering agents. Corneal endothelial cell loss is a rare complication but should be considered in patients with pre-existing corneal conditions. An additional potential complication is the development of glare or visual disturbances, particularly if the iridotomy is large or positioned near the visual axis. Understanding this, the iridotomy location is usually targeted for the superior peripheral iris, which is covered by the upper lid to help negate this possibility.

In some cases, the iridotomy may close over time necessitating a repeat procedure. This closure can occur due to the formation of fibrotic iris tissue over the iridotomy site, particularly in younger patients or those with thicker irides. Regular follow-up is essential to assess for continued patency and ensure long-term efficacy.

Chapter 9
Surgical Approaches

Surgical Interventions

Surgical interventions become necessary when pharmacologic therapies and laser treatments fail to adequately control intraocular pressure, or when there is evidence of disease progression despite maximal medical management. The goal of surgery in glaucoma is to create new drainage pathways for aqueous humor or to enhance existing ones, thereby lowering IOP and preventing further optic nerve damage. The most common surgical procedures include trabeculectomy, implantation of glaucoma drainage devices, and various forms of minimally invasive glaucoma surgery (MIGS).

Trabeculectomy

Trabeculectomy is the most widely performed glaucoma surgery and is considered the gold standard for IOP reduction in patients with advanced or refractory glaucoma. The procedure involves the creation of a new drainage pathway which allows aqueous to bypass the trabecular meshwork and exit the eye, thereby lowering IOP.

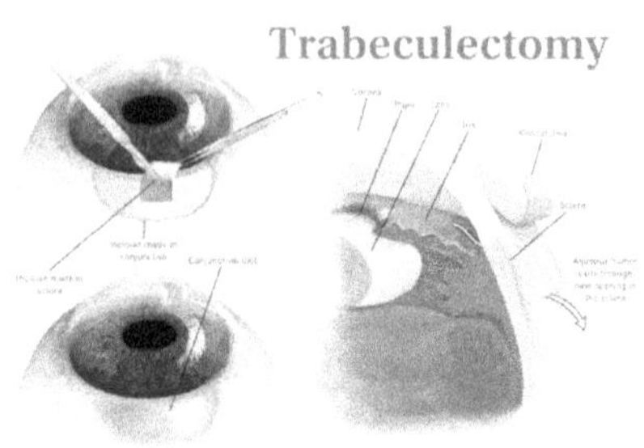

Trab Technique

During trabeculectomy, a partial-thickness scleral flap is created, and a small fistula is made into the anterior chamber of the eye. This fistula *permits aqueous to drain from the anterior chamber into a subconjunctival bleb*, a reservoir formed under the conjunctiva, where aqueous is absorbed by surrounding tissues. The scleral flap is sutured to regulate flow of aqueous humor, preventing excessively low IOP or hypotony while ensuring adequate drainage.

To minimize the risk of scarring and subsequent failure of the bleb, antifibrotic agents such as mitomycin-C or 5-fluorouracil (5-FU) are frequently applied during surgery. These agents inhibit fibroblast proliferation and reduce the likelihood of bleb failure caused by excessive scarring, which is a common cause of long-term surgical failure.

Trabeculectomy is indicated for patients with advanced glaucoma who have not achieved adequate IOP control with medical therapy or laser treatments. It is also suitable for patients with primary open-angle glaucoma, angle-closure glaucoma, and various secondary glaucomas where other interventions have failed.

The efficacy of trabeculectomy is well-documented, with success rates ranging from 60% to 90% depending on the criteria for success and the patient population. The procedure typically reduces IOP by 30-50% from baseline levels and can potentially eliminate the need for glaucoma medications in some patients. However, the success of trabeculectomy is influenced by factors such as patient age, presence of ocular inflammation, and the exact surgical technique employed.

While trabeculectomy is effective, it is associated with a range of potential complications. Early postoperative complications include hypotony, shallow anterior chamber, choroidal effusion, and/or hyphema. Hypotony can lead to serious complications such as corneal decompensation, maculopathy, and suprachoroidal hemorrhage, all of which can compromise final outcomes. Meticulous surgical technique and vigilant postoperative management are essential to minimize risk of these complications.

Late complications of trabeculectomy often involve bleb-related issues, such as bleb leaks, blebitis, and endophthalmitis. Bleb leaks can result in hypotony and increase the risk of infection, while infectious blebitis or endophthalmitis are severe and require prompt treatment with antibiotics or surgical intervention.

Another significant concern is long-term failure of the trabeculectomy due to scarring and fibrosis of the bleb, which can lead to a gradual increase in IOP over time. This is particularly common in younger patients, those with a history of ocular inflammation, or those who have undergone previous surgery. Regular and frequent follow-up is key to monitor for signs of bleb failure and manage any complications that may arise.

Glaucoma Drainage Devices

Glaucoma drainage devices (GDDs), also known as *tube shunts or setons*, are surgical implants used to lower intraocular pressure in patients with glaucoma by *diverting aqueous from the anterior chamber to an external reservoir, typically located beneath the conjunctiva*. GDDs are particularly useful in cases where trabeculectomy is unlikely to succeed or has previously failed, as well as in patients with complex or refractory glaucoma, where traditional surgical methods may be compromised by factors such as fibrosis or inflammation.

There are two main types of GDDs, valved and non-valved devices. Valved devices, such as the *Ahmed Glaucoma Valve*, feature a built-in mechanism which controls the flow of aqueous preventing excessive drainage and minimizing risk of early postoperative hypotony. In contrast, non-valved devices such as the *Baerveldt and Molteno implant*s do not have an intrinsic flow-control mechanism. As a result, these devices require a staged surgical approach or temporary occlusion of the tube to prevent hypotony in the early postoperative period. Each device has its own advantages and limitations, with the choice often tailored to the individual patient's needs and the surgeon's experience.

Implantation involves placing a *silicone tube into the anterior chamber of the eye, with the other end of the tube connected to a reservoir plate*. This plate is positioned beneath the conjunctiva, where it eventually becomes encapsulated by fibrous tissue forming a filtration bleb. This bleb allows the aqueous to be absorbed by surrounding tissues thereby lowering IOP.

The surgical technique varies depending on the type of device used, but precise placement of the tube is critical to avoid complications such as damage to the corneal endothelium, iris, or lens. The tube is typically secured with sutures, and in many cases, the exposed portion of the tube is covered with a patch graft made of donor sclera, pericardium, or another biocompatible material to reduce risk of erosion through the conjunctiva which could lead to infection or endophthalmitis.

GDDs are indicated for individuals with refractory glaucoma who have not achieved adequate IOP control with medical therapy, laser treatments, or trabeculectomy. They are particularly beneficial in cases of neovascular glaucoma, uveitic glaucoma, and other secondary glaucomas where significant scarring or inflammation may compromise the success of a trabeculectomy. They are also used in pediatric glaucoma and in eyes that have undergone multiple previous surgeries, for which other surgical options are limited.

John R Martinelli MD OD FAAO

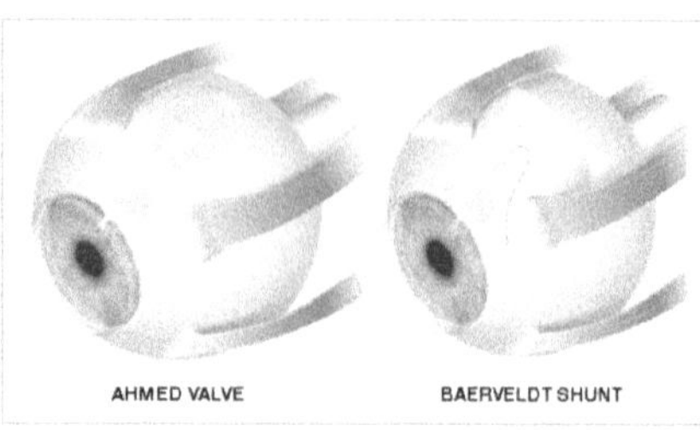

Glaucoma Drainage Devices

They are generally effective in lowering IOP with success rates comparable to or slightly lower than those of trabeculectomy, depending on the patient population and the type of device used. Valved devices are associated with a lower risk of early postoperative hypotony due to their flow-control mechanism, but they may have higher long-term failure rates due to the potential for development of encapsulated blebs which can resist fluid flow. Non-valved devices tend to provide more sustained IOP reduction over the long-term but carry a higher risk of early postoperative complications, particularly hypotony.

Despite their efficacy, GDDs are associated with a range of potential complications in addition to hypotony. Other postoperative complications include tube migration or retraction, tube exposure, corneal endothelial damage, or encapsulation of the reservoir plate which can impede the device's ability to lower intraocular pressure. In some cases, additional surgery may be required to manage these complications or place a second GDD if the first fails.

Long-term complications include erosion of the conjunctiva over the tube, which can expose the tube to the external environment increasing risk of infection and potentially leading to conditions such as endophthalmitis. Chronic contact between the tube and the corneal endothelium can also result in progressive corneal decompensation, which may ultimately necessitate corneal transplantation. Regular follow-up is therefore essential to monitor for these possible complications.

Minimally Invasive Glaucoma Surgery

Minimally invasive glaucoma surgery encompasses a variety of surgical procedures designed to lower intraocular pressure with less trauma and fewer complications compared to traditional glaucoma procedures like trabeculectomy or glaucoma drainage device implantation. MIGS procedures are characterized by their use of *small incisions, minimal disruption to ocular tissues, and a faster recovery time*, making them an attractive option for individuals with mild to moderate glaucoma. The primary goal is to enhance outflow of aqueous humor thereby lowering IOP.

MIGS Procedures

MIGS can be broadly categorized based on their mechanism of action. They can enhance outflow through the trabecular meshwork or bypass the trabecular meshwork entirely.

- **Trabecular Outflow Enhancement**

Procedures utilizing the *iStent*, *Trabectome*, and *Kahook Dual Blade* which are designed to enhance aqueous outflow through the trabecular meshwork. The iStent, for instance, is a tiny titanium device implanted into the trabecular meshwork to create a new channel for aqueous to flow into Schlemm's canal bypassing areas of resistance. The Trabectome ablates a portion of the trabecular meshwork to remove any obstruction or resistance, while the Kahook Dual Blade excises a strip of the trabecular meshwork, both aiming to reduce IOP by improving outflow.

- **Suprachoroidal Shunts**

Suprachoroidal shunts are devices such as the *CyPass Micro-Stent* which were developed to create new drainage pathways by shunting aqueous from the anterior chamber to the suprachoroidal space. The CyPass Micro-Stent, however, was voluntarily withdrawn from the market due to concerns about long-term safety, specifically the risk of corneal endothelial cell loss over time. This emphasizes the importance of ongoing evaluation and monitoring of new devices for potential long-term complications.

- **Subconjunctival Filtration**

An example is the *XEN Gel Stent*. This is a small gelatin-based implant which creates a permanent subconjunctival drainage pathway, similar to a trabeculectomy, but with a lower risk of complications. The XEN stent is designed to lower IOP by diverting aqueous humor from the anterior chamber to a subconjunctival bleb where it is absorbed by surrounding tissues. This approach combines the efficacy of traditional filtration surgery with the safety profile of MIGS.

MIGS procedures are indicated for patients with mild to moderate glaucoma who require IOP reduction but are either not candidates for or wish to avoid traditional glaucoma surgeries. MIGS is also increasingly used in combination with cataract surgery in individuals with coexisting glaucoma, providing the opportunity to address both conditions simultaneously with a single surgical intervention.

While MIGS generally provides more modest IOP reduction compared to trabeculectomy or glaucoma drainage device implantation, it is associated with lower risk of complications and faster recovery times. The efficacy of MIGS varies depending on the type of procedure and the patient population, but it is particularly well-suited for individuals with early-stage glaucoma, those with significant ocular surface issues, or individuals who have difficulty adhering to medical therapy. The minimally invasive nature of MIGS makes it a preferred option for patients seeking a balance between safety and efficacy. Immediate postoperative management typically includes the use of topical corticosteroids to reduce inflammation and prophylactic topical antibiotics. Cycloplegic agents may also be used to maintain pupil dilation and prevent formation of synechiae.

The complications associated with MIGS are rare and generally less severe than those seen with traditional glaucoma procedures. Possible postoperative complications include device malposition which may require surgical revision, and/or insufficient IOP reduction necessitating additional surgery or use of adjunctive pharmacologic therapy. Regarding hypotony, the risk is lower with MIGS than with traditional procedures but can still occur, particularly with devices which bypass the trabecular meshwork entirely. Treatment options may include adjusting the tension of a trabecular meshwork-based device or using viscoelastic agents to stabilize the anterior chamber. In addition, device contact with the corneal endothelium leading to cell loss may trigger corneal decompensation, necessitating additional surgery or endothelial grafts.

MIGS represents a significant advancement in the surgical management of glaucoma, offering a safer less invasive alternative to traditional surgeries with a more favorable recovery profile. While it generally results in less dramatic IOP reduction, lower complication rates and quicker recovery times make this a popular choice for many individuals, particularly in the early-stages or those seeking to avoid risks associated with more invasive surgery.

Surgical Innovations on the Horizon

Glaucoma surgery is poised for significant advancements with the introduction of innovative technologies designed to enhance precision, safety, and efficacy. Among these, robot-assisted surgery and tissue-engineered drainage devices are at the forefront offering new treatment possibilities.

- **Robot-Assisted**

One of the most promising developments is the use of robotic systems to perform delicate procedures with unprecedented precision and stability. The *Preceyes Surgical System*, for instance, represents a major leap forward in this area enabling surgical manipulation with a *precision that is 20-fold greater than that of conventional manual surgery*, achieving movements as fine as sub-5 μm. Originally developed for vitreoretinal surgeries, this system is now being adapted for anterior segment procedures including those for glaucoma.

Robot-assisted offers several key advantages over traditional manual techniques. The micron-level motion precision and tremor stabilization provided by robotic systems allow surgeons to perform intricate procedures with minimal tissue trauma. This high degree of precision is particularly beneficial in glaucoma micro-surgery. Preclinical studies have demonstrated the feasibility of robot-assisted procedures such as trabecular meshwork bypass, goniotomy, and stent implantation in synthetic eye models, suggesting these advancements could lead to improved surgical outcomes and a reduction in postoperative complications.

- **Tissue-Engineered Drainage Devices**

In parallel with robotic advancements, tissue-engineered drainage devices are showing great promise as a sustainable and biocompatible solution for managing elevated intraocular pressure. These devices are designed to *mimic natural drainage pathways of the eye*, thereby reducing IOP while minimizing the risk of complications associated with traditional implants.

Recent preclinical studies have explored various materials, with *collagen-based scaffolds* and *gelatin methacryloyl (GelMA) hydrogels* emerging as particularly promising candidates. A collagen-based scaffold has demonstrated sustained IOP reduction in animal models, highlighting its potential as a long-term solution. Similarly, GelMA hydrogels have shown tunable properties which allow for customization of the device to meet individual patient needs. These hydrogels also promote the formation of capillary-like structures, which could enhance biocompatibility and integration with the host tissue, further improving its efficacy and longevity.

- **Laser-Based MIGS**

Laser-based micro-incision glaucoma surgery techniques have also gained prominence in recent years, offering less invasive options for pressure reduction. These procedures utilize advanced laser technology to create precise incisions or ablations in the trabecular meshwork or other structures involved in aqueous outflow.

Examples of laser-based MIGS include *excimer laser trabeculostomy* (ELT) and *endoscopic cyclophotocoagulation* (ECP). ECP is particularly noteworthy for its ability to target the ciliary body to reduce aqueous humor production. This technique has had favorable results across various types of glaucoma, including mild to moderate cases, refractory glaucoma, and pediatric glaucoma. ECP works by ablating the ciliary processes thereby decreasing aqueous production and subsequently lowering IOP.

Clinical outcomes for ECP are noteworthy. In patients using one glaucoma medication, ECP has been associated with a pressure reduction of approximately 35%. When combined with phacoemulsification, it has demonstrated a 20% reduction in pressure in about 60% of patients, with a success rate of 43% in pediatric patients. These results underscore ECP as a versatile and effective treatment option for a broad spectrum of patients.

Surgical Drug Delivery: 3D Printing & Stimuli-Responsive Systems

The integration of *3D printed ocular inserts* technology into the science of ocular drug delivery represents a significant leap forward, with the potential to revolutionize the way therapies are administered for conditions such as glaucoma. Traditional methods of ocular drug delivery often face challenges related to patient adherence, systemic side effects, and the limited bioavailability of drugs applied topically. By enabling the fabrication of personalized implants and drug delivery systems, 3D printing offers a highly precise and customizable approach which can overcome many of these limitations.

This technology allows for the creation of patient-specific ocular inserts which can be designed to *fit unique anatomical features* of an individual's eye, ensuring optimal placement and effectiveness. It enables the production of implants with customizable complex geometries and structures that can *incorporate multiple therapeutic agents, tailored release profiles, and even sensors to monitor treatment efficacy*. The ability to fabricate personalized drug delivery devices means treatment can be precisely targeted to the needs of each patient, potentially reducing the frequency of dosing, minimizing adverse effects, and enhancing overall treatment outcomes.

For glaucoma therapy, ocular inserts can be engineered to provide sustained and controlled release of prostaglandin analogs, beta-blockers, or carbonic anhydrase inhibitors. These inserts can be implanted into the conjunctival sac or directly onto the ocular surface, delivering medication over extended periods and eliminating the need for daily eye drops. The customization afforded by 3D printing also opens the door to the integration of multiple drugs within a single device, addressing the multifactorial nature of glaucoma and greatly improving management.

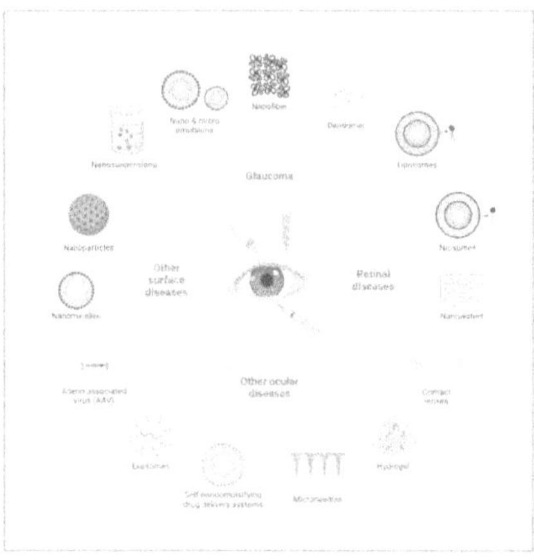

Ocular Drug Delivery

In parallel with advancements in 3D printing, *stimuli-responsive drug release systems* have emerged as a cutting-edge approach to achieving controlled and targeted drug delivery. These systems are designed to *respond to specific physiological stimuli* such as temperature, pH, or ion concentration, triggering the release of therapeutic agents at a desired site within the eye. Such precise control over drug release is particularly valuable in the treatment of glaucoma, where maintaining consistent IOP reduction is critical to preventing progression.

Among the various types of stimuli-responsive systems, *thermo-responsive in situ gelling systems* have gained significant attention. These systems undergo a solution-to-gel transition upon contact with the eye's physiological temperature, allowing the drug-loaded solution to form a gel which adheres to the ocular surface. This gel serves as a reservoir for the sustained release of medication, enhancing both the bioavailability and therapeutic efficacy of the drug. *Poloxamers and poly(N-isopropylacrylamide)/PNIPAAM* are two of the most used polymers in these systems due to their well-characterized thermo-responsive properties and biocompatibility.

Research has demonstrated the effectiveness of thermo-responsive in situ gels for the delivery of various glaucoma medications, including *latanoprost*, *bimatoprost*, and *timolol maleate*. These gels have been shown to provide prolonged drug release, maintaining therapeutic drug levels in the eye over extended periods and reducing the frequency of administration required. The use of such systems not only improves the convenience of glaucoma therapy but also enhances patient adherence, which is often a challenge with traditional eye drop regimens.

Furthermore, the ability to precisely control the gelation process and drug release kinetics through the manipulation of polymer composition and environmental conditions allows for optimization of treatment outcomes. For example, by adjusting the concentration of PNIPAAM in the formulation, researchers can fine-tune the temperature at which gelation occurs and the rate at which the drug is released. This level of control is particularly advantageous in tailoring therapies to the individual needs of patients with varying severities of glaucoma.

The combination of 3D printing and stimuli-responsive drug release systems is defining a new era in ocular drug delivery. By enabling the creation of personalized patient-specific implants with precisely controlled drug delivery systems, these advancements offer the promise of more effective, convenient, and tailored treatments. As research continues to evolve, it is likely these groundbreaking approaches will become integral components of glaucoma therapy.

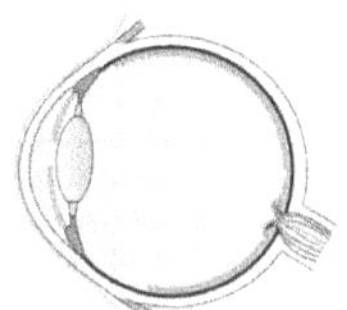

Chapter 10
Genetics & Personalized Glaucoma

Personalized Management

This paradigm shift towards personalized approaches tailoring diagnosis and treatment to individual patients includes genetic profiling, artificial intelligence, and 3D printing, all of which are at the forefront of this revolution.

- **Genetic profiling** has emerged as a powerful tool for risk stratification and treatment selection in glaucoma. A recent study demonstrated individuals in the *top decile of genetic risk are at a 15-fold increased likelihood* of developing advanced glaucoma compared to those in the bottom decile. By identifying high-risk patients through genetic screening, we can implement more intensive management and early intervention strategies. Moreover, genetic information can guide selection of targeted therapies based on an individual's unique molecular profile.

- **AI** is a transformative technology with machine learning algorithms analyzing vast amounts of clinical data, including imaging and visual field results, resulting in *greater predictive ability of an individual's risk of progression and response to treatment*. A deep learning model developed by Thakur et al. achieved an impressive area under the curve of 0.95 in diagnosing glaucoma and 0.88 and 0.77 for forecasting the condition 1 to 3 years and 4 to 7 years before onset, respectively. Such predictive models can dictate personalized treatment plans and optimize follow-up intervals based on an individual's unique risk profile.

- **3D printing** is also revolutionizing the development of patient-specific glaucoma drainage devices. Traditional glaucoma drainage implants, while effective, are designed for the average eye and may not account for individual variations in ocular anatomy. 3D printing enables the fabrication of customized implants which *conform precisely to an individual's unique ocular structures*, potentially improving surgical outcomes and reducing complications. A recent study demonstrated the feasibility of 3D printing patient-specific glaucoma drainage devices using biocompatible materials, paving the way for personalized surgical interventions.

Tailoring diagnosis and treatment based on the unique individual defines personalized glaucoma management. Genetics, family history, age, central corneal thickness, axial length, optic nerve, IOP and others all influence both the likelihood of developing glaucoma and the rate of progression. By *stratifying patients based on their risk profile*, we can implement more intensive monitoring and early intervention for high-risk individuals while adopting a more conservative approach for those at lower risk. This strategy not only improves patient outcomes but also reduces the burden of unnecessary interventions.

Genetic Profiling

Genetic pre-screening for glaucoma, as exemplified by population-based initiatives like the EyeLife study, holds tremendous potential for identifying individuals at heightened risk of developing glaucoma and tailoring their management strategies accordingly. By employing a meticulously curated *glaucoma genetic risk score* (GRS) derived from genome-wide significant single nucleotide polymorphisms associated with glaucoma and its related endophenotypes, researchers aim to refine current SNP-based glaucoma risk prediction models. The ultimate goal is to apply these models prospectively as a pre-screening tool in clinical practice. If successful, genetic pre-screening could enhance the efficiency and effectiveness of glaucoma screening programs by focusing resources on high-risk individuals, potentially preserving vision and improving quality of life for millions globally.

- **Genetic Factors**

Mutations in specific genes have been directly linked to different forms of glaucoma, providing a pathway for more precise diagnostic and therapeutic approaches. For instance, mutations in the *MYOC gene* are associated with 3-4% of primary open-angle glaucoma cases, particularly those characterized by elevated intraocular pressure. These MYOC variants often lead to a form of glaucoma that may not respond well to conventional medical treatments, necessitating early surgical intervention. Similarly, mutations in the *OPTN and TBK1 genes* are associated with 1-3% of normal-tension glaucoma cases, where optic nerve damage occurs despite normal IOP levels.

Genetic testing is currently recommended for patients with juvenile-onset open-angle glaucoma, congenital glaucoma, and may be considered in those with a strong family history of glaucoma. Identifying these genetic mutations allows for the implementation of personalized treatment strategies, including earlier intervention and more rigorous surveillance for affected individuals and their families. This approach not only optimizes treatment efficacy but also enables more targeted monitoring, which is crucial for preventing disease progression.

- **Gene Therapy**

Gene therapy represents a promising frontier in glaucoma treatment, offering the potential to address the underlying genetic causes of the disease. By *delivering therapeutic genes directly to specific ocular cells*, gene therapy aims to provide long-term neuroprotection and reduce IOP, thereby altering the course of glaucoma. *Adeno-associated viruses (AAVs) vectors* have emerged as the most widely used vectors for gene delivery to retinal ganglion cells due to their high transfection efficiency and low immunogenicity. Notably, intravitreal injection of AAV serotype 2 (AAV2) has demonstrated an RGC transfection efficiency of approximately 85%, with sustained gene expression lasting over seven months.

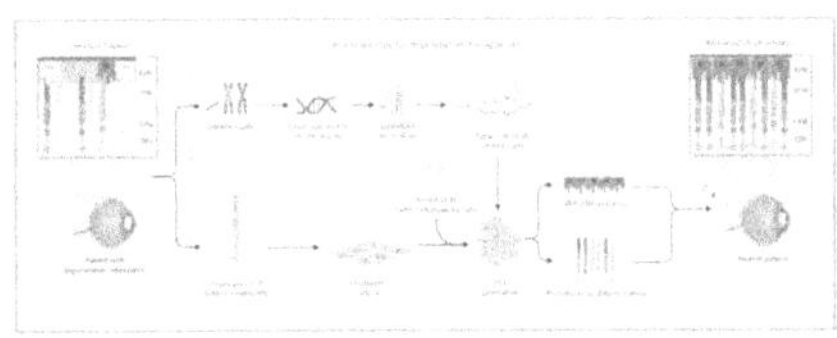

Regenerative Cellular Therapy

Researchers are exploring various gene therapy targets, including growth factors such as *brain-derived neurotrophic factor* (BDNF) which promotes the survival of RGCs, and *apoptosis regulators like Bcl-xL*, which inhibit cell death pathways. Additionally, gene therapy approaches are being developed to enhance the expression of *IOP-lowering receptors*, such as the *prostaglandin F2α receptor* within the eye. Although still in the early stages of clinical development, gene therapy holds immense promise for providing targeted and sustained therapeutic effects in glaucoma management, potentially revolutionizing the way this condition is treated.

- **Pharmacogenomics**

As the field of glaucoma therapeutics continues to evolve, the concept of personalized medicine is becoming increasingly relevant. By tailoring treatment strategies to an individual's unique genetic profile, risk factors, and disease characteristics, we can optimize therapeutic efficacy and improve patient outcomes. Pharmacogenomics, *the study of how genes influence an individual's response to drugs*, plays a key role in this approach.

Genetic variations in drug-metabolizing enzymes, transporters, and receptors can significantly influence the efficacy and safety of glaucoma medications. For example, *polymorphisms in the CYP2D6 gene* have been associated with variable responses to timolol, a commonly prescribed beta-blocker. By genotyping patients for relevant polymorphisms, clinicians can select the most appropriate medication and dosage, thereby minimizing side effects and maximizing therapeutic benefits. Similarly, *mutations in the MYOC and OPTN genes* may influence the response to prostaglandin analogs, which are widely used to lower IOP in glaucoma patients.

As personalized treatment strategies in glaucoma management continue to gain traction, it is very important to validate their clinical utility through appropriate studies and ensure accessibility to all patients who can benefit from them. By using the power of pharmacogenomics, risk stratification, and precision medicine, glaucoma care is poised to enter this new era where treatment is more precisely tuned into the unique characteristics of each person. This personalized approach holds immense promise for preserving vision and improving the quality of life for millions of individuals affected by this sight-threatening condition worldwide.

Chapter 11
Regenerative Medicine & Glaucoma

The science of regenerative medicine provides exciting advances, offering innovative approaches in vision restoration by *replacing lost retinal ganglion cells and regenerating the optic nerve*. Current therapies focus on lowering intraocular pressure but cannot reverse neuropathic and retinal damage already incurred. Regenerative strategies, including RGC transplantation, optic nerve regeneration techniques, and tissue engineering for the trabecular meshwork are emerging as potential game-changers.

Retinal Ganglion Cell Transplantation

RGC transplantation aims to replace neurons lost due to glaucomatous damage, thereby restoring visual function. *Stem cell-derived RGCs* have shown promise as a viable source for transplantation, with studies demonstrating their ability to integrate into the host retina and establish synaptic connections. However, several challenges must be overcome including low graft survival rates, limited migration and integration of transplanted cells, and need for immunosuppression to prevent rejection.

Researchers are exploring various strategies to enhance survival and integration of transplanted RGCs. Co-transplantation with supportive cell types, such as Müller glia or mesenchymal stem cells, has been shown to improve graft survival and provide axonal support. Additionally, the use of biomaterials and scaffolds can provide a favorable microenvironment for transplanted cells facilitating their integration and survival.

Optic Nerve Regeneration Techniques

Regenerating the optic nerve is considered the "holy grail" of restoring visual function in glaucoma and many other optic neuropathies. The optic nerve, composed of RGC axons, exhibits very limited regenerative capacity in mammals. However, recent advances in understanding molecular mechanisms underlying axon regeneration have paved way for novel and exciting therapeutic approaches.

One promising strategy involves *modulating the intrinsic growth capacity of RGC axons*. The manipulation of key signaling pathways, such as the mTOR and PTEN pathways, has been shown to promote axon regeneration of the optic nerve in animal models. Additionally, the use of neurotrophic factors such as brain-derived neurotrophic factor and ciliary neurotrophic factor (CNTF) can support RGC survival and axon growth.

Another approach focuses on *overcoming the inherent inhibitory environment* of optic neuropathy. Glial fibrosis which can form within the nerve contains growth-inhibitory molecules, such as chondroitin sulfate proteoglycans (CSPGs) which hinder axon regeneration. Enzymatic digestion of CSPGs using chondroitinase ABC has also been shown to promote axon regeneration and functional recovery in animal models.

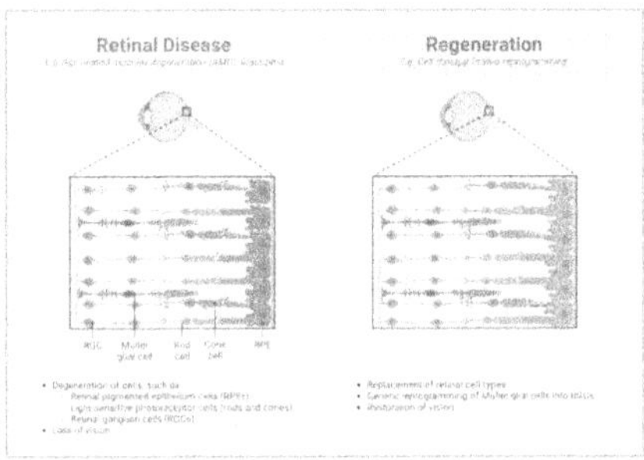

Retina & Optic Nerve Regeneration

Tissue Engineering the Trabecular Meshwork

Pathological changes in the trabecular meshwork (TM), including cellular loss, extracellular matrix remodeling, and reduced phagocytic activity, result in impaired aqueous humor outflow. This dysfunction leads to elevated IOP, a primary risk factor for retinal ganglion cell damage and subsequent vision loss. As current treatments primarily focus on lowering IOP through pharmacologic or surgical means, tissue engineering offers a novel and promising approach to directly address underlying TM dysfunction by regenerating or replacing compromised TM tissue.

One of the most promising strategies in TM tissue engineering involves the use of stem cell-derived TM cells for transplantation. Recent advances have demonstrated *human induced pluripotent stem cells (hiPSCs) can be differentiated into functional TM cells.* These hiPSC-derived TM cells exhibit morphological and physiological characteristics similar to those of native TM cells, including the ability to regulate aqueous humor outflow. In preclinical studies transplantation of hiPSC-derived TM cells into animal models of glaucoma has shown promising results, with transplanted cells successfully integrating into the host TM enhancing aqueous humor outflow and ultimately reducing IOP. This approach holds potential to not only alleviate elevated IOP but also restore normal function to the TM, thereby addressing a common source of ocular hypertension and open angle glaucoma.

Chapter 12

Coexisting Medical Conditions

Glaucoma & Comorbidities: Diabetes, Hypertension, & Others

Glaucoma often coexists with underlying medical conditions such as diabetes mellitus, hypertension, and cardiovascular disease, which are additional considerations in both diagnosis and management. These comorbidities cannot only influence the pathophysiology of glaucoma but also affect the choice of treatment and overall prognosis.

Diabetes Mellitus

Diabetes mellitus is associated with an increased risk of developing glaucoma, particularly primary open-angle glaucoma. The exact mechanisms linking diabetes and glaucoma are not fully understood, but hyperglycemic-induced *vasculopathy, oxidative stress, and neuroinflammation* are believed to play roles. Individuals with diabetes are also more likely to develop secondary glaucoma, such as neovascular glaucoma due to proliferative diabetic retinopathy.

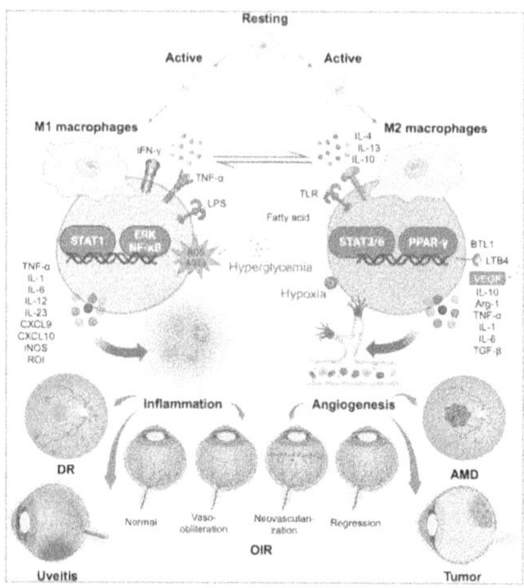

Diabetic Immunopathology

The management of glaucoma in diabetic patients is complicated by the need to control both IOP and blood glucose levels. Certain glaucoma medications, particularly oral carbonic anhydrase inhibitors, can indirectly affect blood glucose control and should be used cautiously in diabetes. Additionally, the presence of diabetic retinopathy may influence the choice of surgical intervention, with some procedures carrying a higher risk of exacerbating retinal complications.

Hypertension & Cardiovascular Disease

Hypertension is common, and in glaucoma patients it has been implicated as both a risk factor and potential contributor to progression. However, the relationship between systemic blood pressure and intraocular pressure is complex, with some studies suggesting *nocturnal hypotension* may be more closely associated with glaucomatous optic neuropathy than hypertension, particularly in normal-tension glaucoma scenarios.

Individuals with cardiovascular disease may face additional challenges in glaucoma management, specifically with the use of beta-blockers which can exacerbate heart failure, bradycardia, and other cardiovascular conditions. In such cases, alternative medical management, laser, or surgical options may be necessary to avoid potential complications.

Gut-Eye Axis

A fascinating connection has been found between glaucoma and the human microbiome, opening new avenues for our understanding and potential treatments. The gut-eye axis, a *bidirectional communication system between the gastrointestinal tract and ocular tissues*, has emerged as a likely key player in glaucoma pathogenesis.

Studies have shown gut dysbiosis - an *imbalance in the intestinal microbial community* - may contribute to the development and progression of glaucoma through various mechanisms.

For instance, alterations in gut bacteria can lead to increased production of lipopolysaccharides (LPS), which activate the TLR4 pathway associated with worsening retinal ganglion cell damage and axonal degeneration. Moreover, certain gut microbes produce metabolites like short-chain fatty acids (SCFAs) that can influence intraocular pressure. Notably, butyrate, produced by bacteria in the phylum Firmicutes, has been found to lower intraocular pressures and improve retinal perfusion in mouse models.

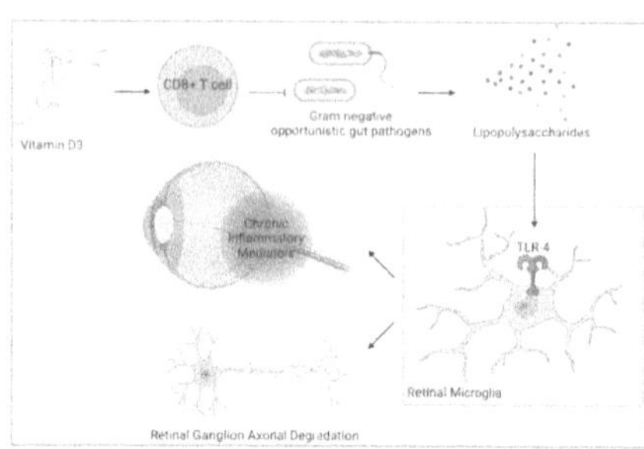

Gut Microbiome & Glaucoma

These discoveries are paving the way for innovative *microbiome-based treatments*. Potential therapeutic strategies include modulating the gut microbiota through dietary interventions, probiotics, or targeted antibiotics to enhance beneficial bacterial populations. Additionally, the administration of specific bacterial metabolites or their analogs could offer new approaches to manage glaucoma progression.

As our understanding of the microbiome-glaucoma relationship deepens, it promises to revolutionize both the diagnosis and treatment of this complex condition, offering hope for more effective, more personalized interventions in the future.

Other Comorbidities

Other medical conditions, such as *chronic obstructive pulmonary disease (COPD), thyroid disease, and autoimmune disorders*, can also impact the management of glaucoma. For example, individuals with COPD may be unable to tolerate beta-blockers due to risk of bronchospasm, necessitating the use of alternative medications. Autoimmune conditions such as rheumatoid arthritis may predispose individuals to uveitic glaucoma, a challenging form of secondary glaucoma which requires careful management of both inflammation and intraocular pressure.

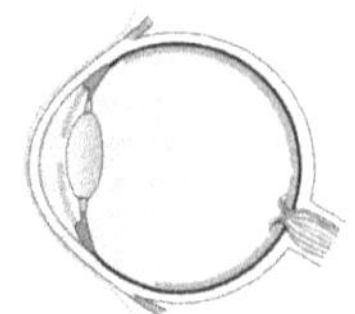

Chapter 13
Case Studies

Glaucoma management is dictated not only by basic science and innovative therapeutic strategies, but also through real-world experience and evidence generated from clinical trials. Clinical trials provide the rigorous data needed to help guide evidence-based practice, while case studies offer valuable insights into the many diverse presentations of glaucoma. However, real-world clinical experience is our ultimate evidence-based data. Only through daily practice can our understanding of diagnoses and management outside of structured and sometimes biased studies be realized. It is through our own personal experience, over years, we gain the critical perspectives necessary to produce successful outcomes and happy patients.

Patient in Your Chair #1

Background: A 57-year-old Caucasian lady with a family history of glaucoma presents for a routine eye examination. She reports no symptoms and has no significant past medical history. Her intraocular pressure is measured at 16 mmHg in both eyes, which is within the normal range. Despite normal IOP, OCT reveals RNFL thinning and optic cupping in both eyes. VF shows a superior arcuate scotoma in the right eye and an early nasal step in the left eye.

Diagnosis: Your diagnosis is normal-tension glaucoma (NTG), a subtype of primary open-angle glaucoma characterized by glaucomatous optic neuropathy despite IOP within normal range. NTG is often associated with vascular risk factors, such as systemic hypotension, which can contribute to optic nerve ischemia.

Management: You start her on brimonidine, an alpha-2 adrenergic agonist, to lower IOP and provide potential neuroprotective effects. She is also advised to monitor her blood pressure, particularly at night, as nocturnal hypotension is a known risk factor for NTG. Lifestyle modifications, including a diet rich in antioxidants and regular exercise are recommended to support overall ocular health.

Outcome: Over the following year, your patient's IOP remains stable at 10 mmHg in each eye with no further progression of her visual field deficits. OCT shows no significant change in RNFL thickness. She continues with regular follow-ups every six months to monitor her IOP, and yearly OCT/VF's to manage any progression.

Discussion: This case highlights the importance of a thorough evaluation in individuals with normal IOP, as NTG can present with significant optic neuropathy and VF defects despite normal pressure. Early diagnosis and management is top priority to prevent further vision loss in NTG, and management involves addressing both IOP and vascular risk factors.

Patient in Your Chair #2

Background: A 68-year-old Asian lady presents to the emergency department with severe ocular pain, headache, and blurred vision in her right eye. She reports seeing halos around lights and has nausea and vomiting. Her medical history includes hypertension controlled with medication. On examination, her right eye is injected and her cornea cloudy. Her pupil is mid-dilated and non-reactive to light. IOP is 48 mmHg in the right eye and 16 mmHg in the left eye.

Diagnosis: You find acute angle-closure, an ophthalmic emergency which occurs when the anterior chamber angle becomes suddenly occluded leading to a rapid rise in IOP.

Management: You treat her with oral acetazolamide and topical IOP-lowering medications, including timolol and brimonidine. Once her IOP is sufficiently lowered, laser peripheral iridotomy is done to create an opening in the peripheral iris and relieve the pupillary block. Prophylactic LPI is also done on her left eye to prevent future angle-closure events.

Outcome: Following treatment, her symptoms rapidly resolve and her IOP stabilizes at 18 mmHg in the right eye and 15 mmHg in the left eye. Her corneal edema clears and her visual acuity returns to baseline. You advise her to continue using topical medications to maintain IOP control, and she is scheduled for regular follow-up visits to monitor for recurrence of angle closure.

Discussion: This case underscores the importance of prompt recognition and treatment of acute angle-closure glaucoma, which can lead to permanent vision loss if not addressed quickly. The use of LPI is critical in both treating the acute event and preventing future episodes in the fellow eye. Individuals with narrow angles should be closely monitored, and prophylactic measures should be considered to reduce the risk of acute angle closure.

Patient in Your Chair #3

Background: A 62-year-old African American man comes to see you with a history of poorly controlled type-2 diabetes mellitus with progressively worsening vision and pain in his right eye. On examination, you find extensive neovascularization of his iris and angle (rubeosis iridis) with an IOP of 44 mmHg. His left eye appears normal with an IOP of 16 mmHg. Retina examination reveals proliferative diabetic retinopathy (PDR) in each eye with extensive neovascularization and vitreous hemorrhage in the right eye.

Diagnosis: Your diagnosis is neovascular glaucoma, a secondary glaucoma caused by growth of abnormal new blood vessels in the anterior chamber angle, typically secondary to ischemic retinal conditions such as in proliferative diabetic retinopathy.

Management: You choose panretinal photocoagulation (PRP) to reduce retinal ischemia and inhibit further neovascularization. Intravitreal injections of anti-VEGF medication, such as bevacizumab, are also administered to target the neovascularization. Topical and oral IOP-lowering medications are prescribed, and a glaucoma drainage tube device is implanted to provide long-term IOP control.

Outcome: Over the following months, your patients neovascularization regresses and his IOP stabilizes at 18 mmHg. His visual acuity remains reduced due to the extent of retinopathy and persistent diabetic macular edema, but he reports significant relief from pain. Continued follow-up is planned to monitor for potential complications such as tube erosion or infection.

Discussion: Neovascular glaucoma is a challenging condition to manage due to its association with severe underlying retinal disease. Early intervention with anti-VEGF therapy and PRP is often beneficial in controlling angle neovascularization and thus reducing IOP. The use of glaucoma drainage devices provides an effective means of long-term IOP control in cases where medical therapy alone is insufficient.

Chapter 14

Key Clinical Trials & Practice Impact

Clinical trials are the backbone of evidence-based medicine, providing research data needed to guide clinical practice and treatment protocols. In glaucoma, numerous landmark trials have shaped our understanding and influenced management of various glaucoma subtypes. Below are key clinical trials and their impact on clinical practice.

Ocular Hypertension Treatment Study

Background: The Ocular Hypertension Treatment Study (OHTS) was a multicenter randomized clinical trial designed to evaluate the effectiveness of topical ocular hypotensive medication in *preventing or delaying the onset of primary open-angle glaucoma* in individuals with elevated intraocular pressure. The study enrolled over 1,600 participants with ocular hypertension, IOP between 24 and 32 mmHg, but no signs of glaucomatous neuropathy.

Findings: OHTS demonstrated treatment with IOP-lowering medications significantly reduced the risk of developing POAG by approximately 50% over a 5-year period. The study also identified several key risk factors for the development of POAG, including older age, higher baseline IOP, thinner central corneal thickness (CCT), and larger vertical cup-to-disc ratio.

Impact on Practice: The findings of OHTS have had a profound impact on the management of ocular hypertension. The study provided *strong evidence for the benefit of early IOP-lowering treatment* in patients at high risk of developing glaucoma. Additionally, the identification of CCT as a significant risk factor led to the widespread adoption of pachymetry in the assessment of glaucoma risk and the interpretation of IOP measurements. OHTS also highlighted the importance of individualized risk assessment in deciding whether to initiate treatment in patients with ocular hypertension.

Early Manifest Glaucoma Trial

Background: The Early Manifest Glaucoma Trial (EMGT) was a randomized clinical trial conducted in Sweden that investigated the effects of *immediate versus delayed treatment* on the progression of early primary open-angle glaucoma. The study enrolled 255 patients with newly diagnosed early POAG and randomized them to either immediate treatment with laser trabeculoplasty and betaxolol or no treatment (observation).

Findings: The EMGT found that immediate treatment significantly reduced the risk of glaucoma progression by approximately 50% over a median follow-up of 6 years. The study also identified baseline factors associated with a higher risk of progression, including higher IOP, older age, and the presence of pseudoexfoliation.

Impact on Practice: The EMGT reinforced the importance of early intervention in the management of POAG. The study provided strong evidence that *lowering IOP, even in patients with early glaucoma, can significantly reduce the risk of disease progression.* These findings have influenced clinical practice by supporting the use of IOP-lowering therapy in patients with early-stage glaucoma and highlighting the importance of regular monitoring to detect progression.

Advanced Glaucoma Intervention Study

Background: The Advanced Glaucoma Intervention Study (AGIS) was a long-term, multicenter clinical trial designed to evaluate the outcomes of different surgical interventions in patients with advanced glaucoma who had failed initial medical therapy. The study *compared the efficacy of trabeculectomy (TRAB) and argon laser trabeculoplasty* as initial surgical treatments, followed by the other procedure if initial treatment failed.

Findings: The AGIS found that both surgical interventions were effective in lowering IOP and slowing the progression of glaucoma, but the *sequence of treatments influenced long-term outcomes.* The study reported that African American patients who underwent initial ALT followed by TRAB had better long-term visual field outcomes compared to those who underwent initial TRAB. In contrast, white patients had similar outcomes regardless of the treatment sequence.

Impact on Practice: The AGIS provided valuable insights into the management of advanced glaucoma, particularly in the context of surgical intervention. The study's findings have influenced clinical decision-making by highlighting the importance of considering patient demographics and individual risk factors when selecting surgical treatments. The AGIS also underscored the need for long-term follow-up and monitoring in patients undergoing glaucoma surgery.

Collaborative Normal-Tension Glaucoma Study

Background: The Collaborative Normal-Tension Glaucoma Study (CNTGS) was a randomized clinical trial that investigated the *effects of IOP-lowering treatment on the progression of normal-tension glaucoma*. The study enrolled patients with NTG and randomized them to either immediate IOP-lowering treatment (targeting a 30% reduction in IOP) or no treatment (observation).

Findings: The CNTGS found that IOP-lowering treatment significantly reduced the risk of glaucoma progression in patients with NTG, particularly in those with more advanced disease or higher baseline IOP. However, the study also reported that a substantial proportion of untreated patients did not experience disease progression over the follow-up period, highlighting the variability in the natural history of NTG.

Impact on Practice: The CNTGS has had a significant impact on the management of NTG by providing evidence that *lowering IOP can be beneficial in reducing the risk of progression*. The study also highlighted the importance of individualized treatment decisions in NTG, with careful consideration of the patient's risk factors and disease severity. The findings of the CNTGS have informed the development of treatment guidelines and have emphasized the need for regular monitoring in patients with NTG.

Tube vs Trabeculectomy Study

Background: The Tube vs Trabeculectomy (TVT) Study was a randomized clinical trial that compared the *long-term outcomes of glaucoma drainage devices and trabeculectomy* with mitomycin C in patients with medically uncontrolled glaucoma who had undergone previous ocular surgery. The study enrolled 212 patients and randomized them to either a GDD (specifically the Baerveldt implant) or TRAB with mitomycin C.

Findings: The TVT Study found both surgical approaches were effective in lowering IOP, but the GDD group had a higher success rate and lower risk of serious complications compared to the TRAB group over a 5-year follow-up period. Patients in the GDD group also required fewer additional glaucoma surgeries and had better long-term IOP control.

Impact on Practice: The TVT Study has influenced clinical practice by providing evidence that GDDs are a *viable and often preferable option for patients with refractory glaucoma*, particularly those who have failed previous trabeculectomy or other surgical interventions. The study's findings have led to an increased use of GDDs in the management of complex glaucoma cases and have informed the development of treatment guidelines for surgical glaucoma management.

Chapter 15

Real World Glaucoma & Long-Term Outcomes

While clinical trials provide valuable data on the efficacy and safety of treatments in controlled environments, real-world evidence and long-term outcomes offer critical insights into how therapies perform in everyday clinical practice.

Real World Evidence

Real-world evidence (RWE) refers to data collected from routine clinical practice, as opposed to controlled settings of clinical trials. RWE provides important insights into *how treatments perform in diverse patient populations, including those with comorbidities, different ethnic backgrounds, and varying levels of disease severity.*

For instance, real-world studies have highlighted the challenges of medication adherence in glaucoma management, with many individuals struggling to maintain consistent use of prescribed eye drops over the long term. Factors such as cost, adverse effects, and the complexity of treatment regimens can all impact adherence leading to suboptimal outcomes. These findings have prompted the development of strategies to improve adherence, such as patient education, simplified dosing regimens, and the use of fixed-dose combination therapies.

RWE has also provided valuable information on the outcomes of newer treatment modalities, such as minimally invasive glaucoma surgery. While clinical trials have demonstrated the safety and efficacy of MIGS, real-world studies have highlighted the variability in outcomes depending on the specific device used, the surgeon's experience, and the patient's baseline characteristics. These findings affect clinical decision-making and have led to the refinement of surgical techniques and patient selection criteria.

Role of Registries & Cohort Studies

Registries and cohort studies are valuable sources of real-world evidence, providing large datasets which can be used to assess long-term outcomes, treatment patterns, and progression. These studies offer the advantage of *capturing data from a wide range of clinical settings and patient populations*, making them more representative of real-world clinical practice.

For example, the *Collaborative Initial Glaucoma Treatment Study* (CIGTS) was a multi-center cohort study which followed over 600 patients with newly diagnosed open-angle glaucoma to compare outcomes of medical versus surgical treatment. The study provided valuable insights into long-term efficacy and safety of treatment approaches and highlighted the importance of individualized treatment decisions based on patient preferences, disease severity, and risk factors.

Similarly, the *United Kingdom Glaucoma Treatment Study* (UKGTS) used a registry-based approach to assess long-term outcomes of various glaucoma treatments in a large diverse population. The study's findings influenced clinical guidelines and have contributed to the development of more personalized treatment strategies in glaucoma management.

Long Term Outcomes

Long-term follow-up studies are essential for understanding the durability of treatment effects and the potential for late complications in management. These studies provide valuable information on the natural history of glaucoma, long-term effectiveness of various interventions, and factors associated with progression.

For example, long-term follow-up of patients in the Advanced Glaucoma Intervention Study (AGIS) revealed while both *trabeculectomy and argon laser trabeculoplasty were effective in lowering IOP, risk of visual field progression remained the same* over time, particularly in patients with higher baseline IOP or more advanced glaucomatous neuropathy. These findings underscore the importance of ongoing management and the potential need for additional interventions in advanced glaucoma.

Similarly, long-term outcomes from the Tube Versus Trabeculectomy Study have shown while *glaucoma drainage devices provide durable IOP control, patients may still require adjunctive therapies* or additional surgeries to maintain target

IOP over time. The risk of complications, such as tube erosion or endophthalmitis, also highlights the need for careful patient selection and postoperative care.

Future of Long-Term Outcomes & Real-World Evidence

As glaucoma management continues to evolve, the importance of long-term outcomes and real-world evidence will only increase. Advances in data collection, including the use of electronic medical records, wearable devices, and patient-reported outcomes will provide more comprehensive and accurate data regarding the long-term impact of various strategies in glaucoma management.

The integration of artificial intelligence and machine learning into the analysis of real-world data will also enhance our ability to identify patterns, predict outcomes, and personalize treatment strategies. By combining data from clinical trials, registries, and real-world practice, we can gain a deeper understanding of the true impact of therapies so to improve quality of care for individuals with this chronic sight-threatening condition.

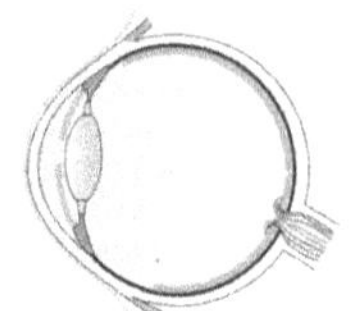

Chapter 16

References & Resources

Books

Glaucoma: A Patient's Guide to the Disease by Mark J. Kupersmith

This book provides an accessible overview of glaucoma, including its causes, symptoms, and treatment options, written for both patients and healthcare providers.

Clinical Glaucoma Management by Shibal Bhartiya

A comprehensive guide focusing on the clinical aspects of glaucoma management, including surgical techniques and the latest advancements in treatment.

The Glaucoma Handbook by James C. Tsai and Thomas R. Yorio

A detailed handbook offering insights into the pathophysiology, diagnosis, and management of glaucoma, with contributions from leading experts in the field.

Essentials of Glaucoma by Malik Y. Kahook and Joel S. Schuman

A practical resource for clinicians, covering the essential aspects of glaucoma diagnosis, treatment, and patient management.

Articles

1. Kooner K, Rehman M, Suresh S, Buchanan E, Albdour MQ, Zuberi H. The role of optical coherence tomography angiography in glaucoma. IntechOpen. 2023. doi:10.5772/intechopen.110272. Available from: https://www.intechopen.com/chapters/86505

2. Ilhan A, Taş A. Indentation tonometry: Schiotz tonometer. 2018. Available from: https://api.semanticscholar.org/CorpusID:54079372

3. Glaucoma [Internet]. EntoKey. Available from: https://entokey.com/glaucoma-27/

4. Gonioscopy [Internet]. Wikipedia. Available from: https://en.wikipedia.org/wiki/Gonioscopy

5. Yang C, Huang X, Li X, Yang C, Zhang T, Wu Q, Liu D, et al. Wearable and implantable intraocular pressure biosensors: recent progress and future prospects. Adv Sci (Weinh). 2021;8(2002971). doi:10.1002/advs.202002971. Available from: https://www.researchgate.net/publication/348666140_Wearable_and_Implantable_Intraocular_Pressure_Biosensors_Recent_Progress_and_Future_Prospects/citation/download

6. Yao Y, Li J, Zhou Y, Wang S, Zhang Z, Jiang Q, Li K. Macrophage/microglia polarization for the treatment of diabetic retinopathy. Front Endocrinol (Lausanne). 2023;14:1276225. doi:10.3389/fendo.2023.1276225. Available from: https://www.frontiersin.org/journals/endocrinology/articles/10.3389/fendo.2023.1276225/full

7. Laser Peripheral Iridotomy (LPI) [Internet]. Available from: https://www.madhuinstruments.com/wp-content/uploads/2016/12/YAG-Iridectomy.jpg

8. Glaucoma Tube Shunts [Internet]. Wills Eye Hospital. Available from: https://www.willseye.org/glaucoma-tube-shunts/

9. Open angle glaucoma. Am Fam Physician. 2003 May 1;67(9):1937-44. Available from: https://www.aafp.org/pubs/afp/issues/2003/0501/p1937.html

10. Gene therapy strategies for glaucoma from IOP reduction to retinal neuroprotection: progress towards non-viral systems [Internet]. Available from: https://www.sciencedirect.com/science/article/abs/pii/S0169409X23000960

11. Glaucoma: management and future perspectives for nanotechnology-based treatment modalities [Internet]. Available from: https://www.sciencedirect.com/science/article/abs/pii/S092809872030436X

12. Restoring the oxidative balance in age-related diseases – an approach in glaucoma [Internet]. Available from: https://www.sciencedirect.com/science/article/pii/S1568163722000149

13. Wireless theranostic smart contact lens for monitoring and control of intraocular pressure in glaucoma [Internet]. Available from: https://www.nature.com/articles/s41467-022-34597-8

14. A prospective analysis of the simplified student sight savers program on open-angle glaucoma cost burden in underserved communities [Internet]. Available from: https://www.researchgate.net/figure/Common-risk-factors-for-developing-glaucoma_fig3_360749143

15. Topical Medication Therapy for Glaucoma and Ocular Hypertension [Internet]. Available from: https://www.frontiersin.org/journals/pharmacology/articles/10.3389/fphar.2021.749858/full

16. Foster PJ, Buhrmann R, Quigley HA, Johnson GJ. The role of intraocular pressure in glaucoma: theories and evidence. Ophthalmology. 2018;125(3):400-408.

17. Huang D, Swanson EA, Lin CP, Schuman JS, Stinson WG, Chang W, et al. Advances in optical coherence tomography for glaucoma diagnosis. J Glaucoma. 2018;27(7):595-603.

18. Weinreb RN, Liebmann JM, Cioffi GA, Crowston JG, Lindsey JD, Medeiros FA, et al. Neuroprotection in glaucoma: current concepts and future directions. Prog Retin Eye Res. 2018;65:77-94.

Illustrations

1. BioRender. Cellular Therapy for Degenerative Retinopathies. 2020. Available from: https://app.biorender.com/biorender-

templates/figures/likes/t-5f29c8905e120f00ad5f68cb-cellular-therapy-for-degenerative-retinopathies

2. Ona S. Ocular Drug Delivery Systems. 2024. Available from: https://app.biorender.com/biorender-templates/figures/likes/t-661435fd44f508deaeda78a3-ocular-drug-delivery-systems

3. BioRender. Glaucoma Drainage Implant. 2024. Available from: https://app.biorender.com/biorender-templates/figures/likes/t-663cd774ff1e642bae6c5f8c-glaucoma-drainage-implant

4. Kim S. Structure of the Retina. 2020. Available from: https://app.biorender.com/biorender-templates/figures/likes/t-5fdba689c542b300a3aeb236-structure-of-the-retina

5. BioRender. Retinal Disease and Regeneration. 2023. Available from: https://app.biorender.com/biorender-templates/figures/likes/t-6489c6cc97c2d53d8d4bae8e-retinal-disease-and-regeneration

6. Stiver M. Human Visual Pathway. 2023. Available from: https://app.biorender.com/biorender-templates/figures/likes/t-652bfc3a7dd86a1754f7fef1-human-visual-pathway

7. Pathan J. Roles of Microglia in Neuroinflammation. 2022. Available from: https://app.biorender.com/biorender-templates/figures/all/t-63a4bc394320eed93210b91b-roles-of-microglia-in-neuroinflammation

Case Studies

American Academy of Ophthalmology (AAO) Clinical Education

The AAO offers a comprehensive collection of case studies, clinical guidelines, and educational resources.

Access here: AAO Clinical Education

Glaucoma Research Foundation - Patient Stories and Case Studies

This resource includes patient stories, case studies, and expert opinions on glaucoma management.

Access here: Glaucoma Research Foundation Case Studies

Medscape Ophthalmology Case Studies

Medscape provides a range of ophthalmology case studies, including those focused on glaucoma, with expert commentary.

Access here: Medscape Ophthalmology Cases

Optometry Times - Clinical Case Studies

Optometry Times offers case studies that focus on optometric management of various ocular conditions, including glaucoma.

Access here: Optometry Times Case Studies

Interactive Visuals and Diagnostic Images

EyeWiki by the American Academy of Ophthalmology

EyeWiki offers detailed articles and images on various ophthalmic conditions, including glaucoma.

Access here: EyeWiki

Webvision: The Organization of the Retina and Visual System

Hosted by the University of Utah, Webvision provides comprehensive, interactive content on the retina and visual pathways, including glaucomatous changes.

Access here: Webvision

Optical Coherence Tomography Atlas - University of Iowa

This atlas provides a collection of OCT images, including those showing glaucomatous damage.

Access here: OCT Atlas

Review of Optometry - Clinical Images

Review of Optometry provides an extensive library of clinical images and case discussions, including those related to glaucoma diagnosis and management.

Access here: Review of Optometry Clinical Images

Videos of Surgical Techniques and Procedures

American Academy of Ophthalmology - Video Library

The AAO's video library includes a wide range of surgical videos, including those focused on glaucoma procedures.

Access here: AAO Video Library

Eyetube Glaucoma

Eyetube provides a dedicated section for glaucoma surgery videos, covering techniques such as MIGS, trabeculectomy, and laser procedures.

Access here: Eyetube Glaucoma

University of Iowa EyeRounds Video Atlas

This resource includes a video atlas of ophthalmic surgical procedures, including glaucoma surgery.

Access here: EyeRounds Video Atlas

Optometric Management - Clinical Videos

Optometric Management offers videos related to clinical techniques and procedures, including advanced diagnostic and therapeutic approaches in glaucoma.

Access here: Optometric Management Videos

Clinical Trials

Ocular Hypertension Treatment Study (OHTS)

ClinicalTrials.gov Identifier: NCT00000125

A landmark study that evaluated the effectiveness of early treatment in preventing the onset of primary open-angle glaucoma in patients with ocular hypertension.

The Collaborative Normal-Tension Glaucoma Study (CNTGS)

ClinicalTrials.gov Identifier: NCT00000114

A significant clinical trial investigating the impact of lowering intraocular pressure in patients with normal-tension glaucoma.

Conference Proceedings

World Glaucoma Congress Proceedings

A collection of research papers and presentations from the World Glaucoma Congress, offering insights into the latest advancements in glaucoma research and treatment.

ARVO Annual Meeting Abstracts

Abstracts from the Association for Research in Vision and Ophthalmology (ARVO) Annual Meeting, covering the latest research in glaucoma and related fields.

Additional Resources

American Academy of Ophthalmology (AAO) - Glaucoma Resources

Glaucoma Overview

This resource provides comprehensive information on glaucoma, including educational materials, videos, and patient guides.

National Eye Institute (NEI) - Glaucoma Information

Glaucoma Information Page

An authoritative source of information on glaucoma, offering the latest research updates, treatment guidelines, and patient education resources.

Glaucoma Research Foundation

Understanding Glaucoma

A non-profit organization dedicated to advancing research and providing resources for patients and healthcare providers.

Chapter 17

Glossary of Terms

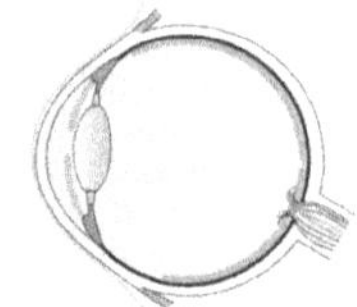

Acanthosis Nigricans

A skin condition characterized by dark, velvety patches in body folds and creases, often associated with insulin resistance and considered a risk factor for diabetes-related eye complications.

Acute Angle-Closure Glaucoma (AACG)

A type of glaucoma characterized by a sudden increase in intraocular pressure (IOP) due to the closure of the anterior chamber angle, leading to an ocular emergency requiring immediate treatment to prevent vision loss.

Angle-Closure Glaucoma (ACG)

A type of glaucoma characterized by the closure of the anterior chamber angle, which leads to a rapid increase in intraocular pressure.

Anterior Chamber

The fluid-filled space inside the eye between the iris and the cornea's innermost surface, known as the endothelium.

Aqueous Humor

A clear, watery fluid that fills the anterior and posterior chambers of the eye, produced by the ciliary body. It provides nutrients to the avascular structures of the eye and maintains intraocular pressure.

Argon Laser Trabeculoplasty (ALT)

A laser procedure used to treat open-angle glaucoma by improving aqueous outflow through the trabecular meshwork, thereby lowering intraocular pressure.

Axenfeld-Rieger Syndrome

A genetic disorder that affects the development of the eyes and other parts of the body, often leading to glaucoma due to anterior segment dysgenesis.

Beta-Adrenergic Antagonists

Also known as beta-blockers, these medications are used to reduce intraocular pressure by decreasing aqueous humor production. Common examples include timolol and betaxolol.

Beta-Blockers

A class of medications used to reduce intraocular pressure by decreasing aqueous humor production.

Bleb

A fluid-filled blister on the eye surface that forms after trabeculectomy surgery, serving as a drainage reservoir for aqueous humor to reduce intraocular pressure in glaucoma patients.

Blepharospasm

An involuntary tight closure of the eyelids, which can be associated with various ocular conditions, including dry eye and anterior segment disease.

Brimonidine

An alpha-2 adrenergic agonist used in the treatment of glaucoma to lower intraocular pressure by decreasing aqueous humor production and increasing uveoscleral outflow.

Ciliary Body

A structure in the eye involved in aqueous humor production and accommodation. It includes the ciliary muscle, which controls lens shape, and the ciliary processes, which secrete aqueous humor.

Central Corneal Thickness (CCT)

A measurement of the thickness of the central cornea, important in assessing glaucoma risk and the accuracy of intraocular pressure readings.

Choroidal Effusion

The accumulation of fluid in the suprachoroidal space, which can occur as a complication of glaucoma surgery or due to other ocular conditions, potentially leading to increased intraocular pressure.

Ciliochoroidal Effusion

An abnormal collection of fluid in the potential space between the ciliary body and the choroid, often seen in the postoperative setting or with uveitis, potentially causing secondary glaucoma.

Corneal Edema

Swelling of the cornea due to fluid accumulation, which can occur after glaucoma surgery or as a result of elevated intraocular pressure, leading to decreased vision.

Corticosteroid-Induced Glaucoma

A form of secondary glaucoma that results from prolonged use of corticosteroids, leading to increased intraocular pressure due to reduced aqueous outflow.

Cribriform Plate

The perforated region of the sclera through which the optic nerve fibers pass, often referred to in relation to the lamina cribrosa, a key site of glaucomatous damage.

Cyclophotocoagulation

A laser treatment used to reduce intraocular pressure in glaucoma by destroying part of the ciliary body to decrease aqueous humor production.

Cycloplegia

Paralysis of the ciliary muscle, resulting in a loss of accommodation. It can be induced pharmacologically during certain eye examinations or treatments and may affect intraocular pressure measurements.

Deep Sclerectomy

A non-penetrating glaucoma surgery designed to lower intraocular pressure by creating a drainage space in the sclera, reducing the need for a full-thickness trabeculectomy.

Diurnal Variation

Fluctuations in intraocular pressure that occur throughout the day. Understanding a patient's diurnal variation is important in diagnosing and managing glaucoma.

Disc Hemorrhage

Bleeding at the optic nerve head, often associated with glaucoma progression, particularly in normal-tension glaucoma. It is considered a risk factor for visual field deterioration.

Endocyclophotocoagulation (ECP)

A surgical procedure that uses a laser to treat the ciliary processes and reduce aqueous humor production, commonly used in conjunction with cataract surgery in glaucoma patients.

Endothelial Cell Count

A measure of the density of endothelial cells on the inner surface of the cornea. A decrease in these cells can occur after certain glaucoma surgeries, leading to corneal decompensation.

Excimer Laser

A type of ultraviolet laser used in refractive eye surgeries, such as LASIK. It is occasionally mentioned in the context of glaucoma for its role in postoperative complications affecting corneal healing.

Exfoliation Syndrome

Also known as pseudoexfoliation, this condition is characterized by the accumulation of fibrillar material in the anterior segment, significantly increasing the risk for secondary glaucoma.

Filtration Surgery

A term that encompasses surgical procedures like trabeculectomy and glaucoma drainage device implantation, aimed at creating new pathways for aqueous humor outflow to lower intraocular pressure.

Gonioscopy

A diagnostic procedure using a specialized contact lens to visualize the anterior chamber angle of the eye, often necessary for diagnosing and managing different types of glaucoma.

Goniosynechiae

Permanent adhesions between the iris and the trabecular meshwork, often associated with chronic angle-closure glaucoma, leading to impaired aqueous humor drainage.

Hyphema

The presence of blood in the anterior chamber of the eye, which can occur as a complication of glaucoma surgery or trauma. It requires careful monitoring as it can lead to increased intraocular pressure.

Hypotony

A condition characterized by abnormally low intraocular pressure, which can occur after glaucoma surgery and lead to complications such as choroidal detachment or maculopathy.

Indocyanine Green Angiography (ICGA)

An imaging technique used to visualize blood flow in the choroid and retina. It can be useful in diagnosing vascular abnormalities in glaucomatous eyes.

Intraocular Pressure (IOP)

The fluid pressure inside the eye, maintained by the balance between aqueous humor production and outflow. Elevated IOP is a major risk factor for the development and progression of glaucoma.

Iris Bombe

A condition where the iris bows forward due to the accumulation of aqueous humor behind it, often leading to angle-closure glaucoma.

Iridocorneal Endothelial Syndrome (ICE)

A spectrum of disorders that includes essential iris atrophy, Chandler syndrome, and Cogan-Reese syndrome, all of which can lead to secondary angle-closure glaucoma.

Juvenile Open-Angle Glaucoma (JOAG)

A form of primary open-angle glaucoma that occurs in younger individuals, typically between the ages of 10 and 35, often associated with genetic mutations such as those in the MYOC gene.

Lamina Cribrosa

A sieve-like structure at the optic nerve head through which retinal ganglion cell axons pass. It is a key site of damage in glaucoma, particularly in cases of elevated intraocular pressure.

Laser Peripheral Iridotomy (LPI)

A laser procedure used to create an opening in the peripheral iris, allowing aqueous humor to flow from the posterior to the anterior chamber, commonly performed to prevent or treat angle-closure glaucoma.

Laser Suture Lysis

A postoperative procedure performed after trabeculectomy, where laser energy is used to cut sutures and enhance the outflow of aqueous humor through the surgical site.

Latanoprost

A prostaglandin analogue used in the treatment of glaucoma, it increases uveoscleral outflow, effectively lowering intraocular pressure with once-daily dosing.

Minimally Invasive Glaucoma Surgery (MIGS)

A group of surgical procedures designed to lower intraocular pressure with less trauma and fewer complications compared to traditional glaucoma surgeries such as trabeculectomy.

Myocilin (MYOC)

A gene associated with primary open-angle glaucoma (POAG). Mutations in this gene can lead to the accumulation of myocilin protein in the trabecular meshwork, obstructing aqueous outflow and increasing intraocular pressure.

Nanophthalmos

A condition characterized by an abnormally small eye, leading to a crowded anterior chamber and a high risk of angle-closure glaucoma.

Neovascular Glaucoma

A secondary glaucoma caused by the growth of new, abnormal blood vessels in the anterior chamber angle, often associated with ischemic retinal conditions like diabetic retinopathy.

Neuroretinal Rim

The edge of the optic nerve head, where nerve fibers converge to form the optic nerve.

Normal -Tension Glaucoma (NTG)

A form of glaucoma where optic nerve damage and visual field loss occur despite normal intraocular pressure levels. It is often associated with vascular factors such as nocturnal hypotension.

Ocular Hypertension

A condition characterized by elevated intraocular pressure without detectable glaucomatous damage. Individuals with ocular hypertension are at increased risk for developing glaucoma.

Ophthalmodynamometry

A technique used to measure blood flow in the central retinal artery and assess ocular perfusion pressure, which is particularly relevant in patients with normal-tension glaucoma.

Optical Coherence Tomography (OCT)

A non-invasive imaging technology that provides high-resolution cross-sectional images of the retina and optic nerve head, essential for diagnosing and monitoring glaucoma.

Optic Nerve Head (ONH)

The visible portion of the optic nerve as it exits the retina. The ONH is the site where glaucomatous damage, such as cupping and thinning of the neuroretinal rim, is typically assessed.

Pachymetry

The measurement of corneal thickness, which is critical for accurate intraocular pressure readings and glaucoma risk assessment, as thinner corneas can lead to underestimation of IOP.

Phacoemulsification

A modern cataract surgery technique that uses ultrasound to emulsify the lens, often performed in conjunction with glaucoma surgery to manage both conditions simultaneously.

Pigment Dispersion Syndrome (PDS)

A condition where pigment granules from the iris disperse into the anterior chamber and trabecular meshwork, leading to increased intraocular pressure and pigmentary glaucoma.

Pilocarpine

A cholinergic agonist used to lower intraocular pressure in glaucoma by increasing aqueous humor outflow through the trabecular meshwork. It is also used to induce miosis during acute angle-closure glaucoma.

Plateau Iris Syndrome

A condition where the iris is abnormally flat, leading to angle closure despite a patent peripheral iridotomy. It is a cause of secondary angle-closure glaucoma.

Prostaglandin Analogues

Medications that increase the outflow of aqueous humor to lower intraocular pressure in glaucoma patients.

Prostaglandin-Associated Periorbitopathy (PAP)

A side effect of prostaglandin analogue use, characterized by deepening of the upper eyelid sulcus, enophthalmos, and orbital fat atrophy, affecting the cosmetic appearance of the eye.

Pseudoexfoliation Syndrome

A systemic condition characterized by the production of abnormal fibrillary material that deposits on the lens, iris, and trabecular meshwork, increasing the risk of secondary open-angle glaucoma.

Retinal Ganglion Cells (RGCs)

Neurons located in the innermost layer of the retina whose axons form the optic nerve. Loss of RGCs is the primary pathological event in glaucoma, leading to optic nerve damage and vision loss.

Retinal Nerve Fiber Layer (RNFL)

The layer of the retina that contains the axons of retinal ganglion cells, which converge to form the optic nerve. RNFL thickness is a key parameter measured in glaucoma diagnosis and monitoring.

Rho Kinase Inhibitors

A class of medications that lower intraocular pressure by enhancing aqueous humor outflow through the trabecular meshwork. They also reduce episcleral venous pressure and may have neuroprotective effects.

Schlemm's Canal

A circular channel in the eye that collects aqueous humor from the trabecular meshwork and drains it into the bloodstream, playing a critical role in maintaining normal intraocular pressure.

Selective Laser Trabeculoplasty (SLT)

A laser treatment for open-angle glaucoma that targets pigmented trabecular meshwork cells, enhancing aqueous outflow and reducing intraocular pressure with minimal tissue damage.

Suprachoroidal Hemorrhage

A rare but serious complication of glaucoma surgery, where blood accumulates between the choroid and sclera, often leading to sudden vision loss and requiring immediate intervention.

Trabeculectomy

A surgical procedure used to treat glaucoma by creating a new drainage pathway for aqueous humor to leave the eye, thus lowering intraocular pressure. It is often considered when medical therapy and less invasive surgeries fail.

Trabeculodysgenesis

A developmental anomaly of the trabecular meshwork, often seen in congenital glaucoma, where the abnormal trabecular architecture leads to impaired aqueous outflow and elevated intraocular pressure.

Trabecular Meshwork

A spongy tissue located at the base of the cornea and iris, responsible for draining aqueous humor from the eye into the Schlemm's canal. Dysfunction of the trabecular meshwork is a primary cause of elevated intraocular pressure in glaucoma.

Uveoscleral Outflow

A secondary pathway for aqueous humor drainage that bypasses the trabecular meshwork, allowing fluid to exit the eye through the uvea and sclera. This pathway is a target for certain glaucoma medications, such as prostaglandin analogues.

Visual Field Index (VFI)

A global metric used in visual field testing to quantify the overall visual field function, expressed as a percentage, where 100% represents a full visual field.

Visual Field Testing

A diagnostic tool used to assess the visual field, particularly the peripheral vision, which is often affected first in glaucoma. Tests such as standard automated perimetry (SAP) are essential for detecting and monitoring glaucomatous damage.

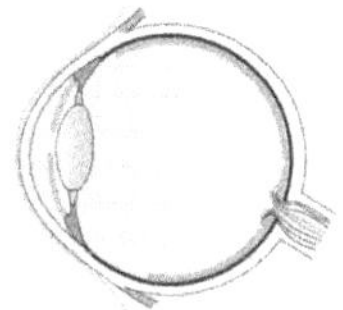

Chapter 18
Q&A

Q: What are the primary differences between primary open-angle glaucoma (POAG) and normal-tension glaucoma (NTG)?

A: POAG is characterized by elevated intraocular pressure (IOP) that damages the optic nerve, leading to visual field loss. NTG, on the other hand, features optic nerve damage and visual field loss despite IOP being within the normal range. NTG is often associated with vascular dysregulation, systemic hypotension, or other factors that compromise optic nerve perfusion.

Q: How does central corneal thickness (CCT) influence the risk and management of glaucoma?

A: CCT affects the accuracy of IOP measurements. A thinner cornea can lead to underestimation of IOP, potentially delaying glaucoma diagnosis. Conversely, a thicker cornea may overestimate IOP, leading to unnecessary treatment. CCT is also an independent risk factor for glaucoma progression.

Q: What are the indications for performing a trabeculectomy in glaucoma patients?

A: Trabeculectomy is indicated in patients with glaucoma who have not achieved adequate IOP control with maximal medical therapy and less invasive surgical options. It is particularly indicated in cases of advanced glaucoma where there is a high risk of vision loss.

Q: What role does the lamina cribrosa play in the pathophysiology of glaucoma?

A: The lamina cribrosa is a sieve-like structure through which retinal ganglion cell axons pass. In glaucoma, increased IOP can deform the lamina cribrosa, leading to mechanical stress and subsequent axonal damage, contributing to optic nerve head cupping and visual field loss.

Q: How does selective laser trabeculoplasty (SLT) compare to argon laser trabeculoplasty (ALT) in the management of open-angle glaucoma?

A: SLT and ALT both aim to improve aqueous outflow through the trabecular meshwork, lowering IOP. SLT uses a lower energy laser, targeting pigmented trabecular cells selectively, which reduces collateral damage and inflammation compared to ALT. SLT is often preferred due to its repeatability and lower risk of side effects.

Q: What are the genetic implications of myocilin (MYOC) mutations in primary open-angle glaucoma?

A: Mutations in the MYOC gene are associated with an autosomal dominant form of juvenile and adult-onset primary open-angle glaucoma. These mutations lead to the accumulation of misfolded myocilin protein in the trabecular meshwork, impairing aqueous outflow and increasing IOP.

Q: What is the significance of optic disc hemorrhages in the progression of glaucoma?

A: Optic disc hemorrhages are a sign of ongoing glaucomatous damage, particularly in NTG. They are associated with a higher risk of visual field progression and may indicate the need for more aggressive IOP-lowering therapy.

Q: How does uveoscleral outflow contribute to intraocular pressure regulation, and what are its clinical implications?

A: Uveoscleral outflow is an alternative pathway for aqueous humor drainage, bypassing the trabecular meshwork. It accounts for a significant portion of aqueous outflow, especially in younger patients. Prostaglandin analogues, which increase uveoscleral outflow, are commonly used in glaucoma management to lower IOP.

Q: What are the clinical challenges in managing neovascular glaucoma, and what treatment strategies are commonly employed?

A: Neovascular glaucoma is challenging due to its association with ischemic retinal diseases, leading to abnormal blood vessel growth in the anterior chamber angle. Treatment involves addressing the underlying retinal ischemia with panretinal photocoagulation or anti-VEGF therapy, along with IOP control using medical therapy and, if necessary, surgical interventions like glaucoma drainage devices.

Q: What factors should be considered when selecting a minimally invasive glaucoma surgery (MIGS) procedure for a patient?

A: Selection of a MIGS procedure depends on factors such as the severity of glaucoma, the patient's IOP target, anatomical considerations (e.g., angle configuration), and whether the patient is undergoing concurrent cataract surgery. MIGS is typically chosen for patients with mild to moderate glaucoma who require moderate IOP reduction.

Q: How do systemic conditions like diabetes and hypertension impact glaucoma management?

A: Diabetes and hypertension can complicate glaucoma management by contributing to ocular blood flow abnormalities, increasing the risk of neovascularization, and affecting the safety and efficacy of certain glaucoma medications. These comorbidities may also necessitate more frequent monitoring and adjustments in treatment.

Q: What is the role of visual field testing in the diagnosis and monitoring of glaucoma?

A: Visual field testing is essential in diagnosing glaucoma and monitoring its progression. It helps detect functional loss in the visual field, particularly in the peripheral vision, which is often the first to be affected in glaucoma. Repeated testing over time is required for assessing disease progression and the effectiveness of treatment.

Q: How does the presence of exfoliation syndrome increase the risk of glaucoma?

A: Exfoliation syndrome is characterized by the production of fibrillar material that accumulates in the anterior segment of the eye, including the trabecular meshwork. This material obstructs aqueous outflow, leading to increased IOP and a higher risk of developing secondary open-angle glaucoma.

Q: What are the potential complications of glaucoma drainage devices (GDDs), and how are they managed?

A: Complications of GDDs include hypotony, tube migration, tube erosion, corneal decompensation, and infection. Management may involve surgical revision, use of bandage contact lenses, and, in some cases, additional procedures to reposition or replace the device.

Q: What is the significance of retinal nerve fiber layer (RNFL) thickness in glaucoma assessment?

A: RNFL thickness, measured by OCT, is a critical indicator of glaucomatous damage. Thinning of the RNFL correlates with the loss of retinal ganglion cells and precedes visual field loss, making it a valuable tool for early diagnosis and monitoring of glaucoma progression.

Q: How do Rho kinase inhibitors work in lowering intraocular pressure in glaucoma patients?

A: Rho kinase inhibitors reduce intraocular pressure by increasing aqueous humor outflow through the trabecular meshwork and reducing episcleral venous pressure. They may also provide neuroprotective effects, making them a promising option for glaucoma management.

Q: What are the clinical indications for performing a laser peripheral iridotomy (LPI)?

A: LPI is indicated in patients with angle-closure glaucoma, those with narrow angles at risk of closure, and individuals with iris bombe. It creates a small hole in the iris, allowing aqueous humor to flow from the posterior to the anterior chamber, relieving pupillary block and reducing IOP.

Q: What is plateau iris syndrome, and how is it managed?

A: Plateau iris syndrome occurs when the peripheral iris is pushed forward, leading to angle closure even after a patent peripheral iridotomy. Management may include laser peripheral iridoplasty to flatten the peripheral iris or additional surgical interventions if necessary.

Q: How does corneal edema affect intraocular pressure measurements in glaucoma patients?

A: Corneal edema, which can result from elevated IOP or post-surgical complications, increases corneal thickness and rigidity, leading to falsely elevated IOP measurements. Accurate assessment may require decongesting the cornea or using alternative tonometry methods.

Q: What is the relevance of gonioscopy in the evaluation of glaucoma?

A: Gonioscopy is an investigation for assessing the anterior chamber angle, determining the type of glaucoma (open vs. closed angle), and identifying anatomical variations or pathologies such as peripheral anterior synechiae, angle recession, or neovascularization, which influence treatment decisions.

Q: How do prostaglandin analogues achieve IOP reduction in glaucoma patients?

A: Prostaglandin analogues lower intraocular pressure by increasing uveoscleral outflow. They are the first-line treatment for most types of glaucoma due to their efficacy, once-daily dosing, and favorable safety profile.

Q: What are the advantages of using OCT angiography (OCTA) in glaucoma management?

A: OCTA provides non-invasive visualization of the retinal and optic nerve head vasculature, allowing for the detection of microvascular changes associated with glaucoma. It helps in identifying early disease, monitoring progression, and evaluating treatment efficacy, especially in normal-tension glaucoma.

Q: What considerations should be taken into account when managing glaucoma in pediatric patients?

A: Pediatric glaucoma management requires careful consideration of the child's age, disease severity, and potential impact on visual development. Surgical intervention is often necessary, and long-term follow-up is critical to monitor for amblyopia, disease progression, and surgical complications.

Q: How does the presence of optic disc cupping correlate with glaucoma progression?

A: Optic disc cupping occurs due to the loss of retinal ganglion cell axons and corresponding loss of neuroretinal rim tissue. Progressive cupping is a hallmark of glaucoma progression and is monitored closely using fundus photography and OCT to guide treatment decisions

Q: What roles do patient education and adherence play in the long-term management of glaucoma?

A: Patient education is vital in ensuring adherence to glaucoma treatment, as the disease is typically asymptomatic until advanced stages. Understanding the importance of consistent medication use, regular follow-up, and lifestyle modifications can significantly impact the long-term outcomes and prevention of vision loss.

Also by Dr. Martinelli

Books:

Dr. Martinelli's Vision & Neurology Casebook: Real-World Insights for Primary Eye Care & Family Medicine

Labs & Imaging for Primary Eye Care

Screens & Vision: Your Eyes in a Digital World

Online:

Dr. Martinelli's Substack: The Fine Art of Patient Management

About the Author

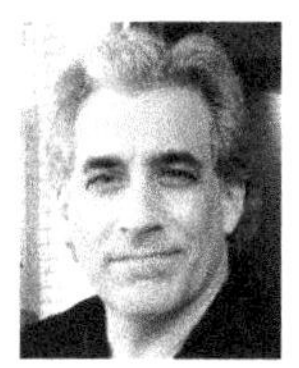

With 27 years on the private practice front lines as an optometric physician prior to earning his medical degree, Dr. Martinelli brings years of extensive clinical experience, combined with medicine, providing rare insight and guidance in the art of patient management.

He offers not theory, but high-yield clinical knowledge to help build practices simply by taking proper care of people, who also happen to be our patients.

Dr. Martinelli is a graduate of St. George's University School of Medicine, Pennsylvania College of Optometry, and Washington & Jefferson College. He is a physician member of the American Medical Association (AMA), American Optometric Association (AOA), and Fellow of the American Academy of Optometry (FAAO).

His clinical articles have been featured over the years in various publications. He very much enjoys teaching, and for more than a decade taught countless students in his practice as a preceptor in ocular disease for the Pennsylvania College of Optometry.

Dr. Martinelli has spoken for Alcon and Allergan, as well as nationally and internationally with topics involving medical eye care, glaucoma, and refractive surgery such as LASIK.

He continues to actively see patients daily in private practice.

Ophthalmic Physician Publishing
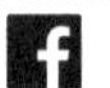  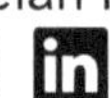 

9 798330 387540